Neuromuscular Junction Disorders

Editors

MAZEN M. DIMACHKIE
RICHARD J. BAROHN

NEUROLOGIC CLINICS

www.neurologic.theclinics.com

Consulting Editor
RANDOLPH W. EVANS

May 2018 • Volume 36 • Number 2

ELSEVIER

1600 John F. Kennedy Boulevard • Suite 1800 • Philadelphia, Pennsylvania, 19103-2899

http://www.theclinics.com

NEUROLOGIC CLINICS Volume 36, Number 2
May 2018 ISSN 0733-8619, ISBN-13: 978-0-323-58368-8

Editor: Stacy Eastman
Developmental Editor: Donald Mumford

Neurologic Clinics (ISSN 0733-8619) is published quarterly by Elsevier Inc., 360 Park Avenue South, New York, NY 10010–1710. Months of issue are February, May, August, and November. Periodicals postage paid at New York, NY, and additional mailing offices. Subscription prices are $312.00 per year for US individuals, $631.00 per year for US institutions, $100.00 per year for US students, $390.00 per year for Canadian individuals, $765.00 per year for Canadian institutions, $423.00 per year for international individuals, $765.00 per year for international institutions, and $210.00 for Canadian and foreign students/residents. To receive student/resident rate, orders must be accompanied by name of affiliated institution, date of term, and the *signature* of program/residency coordinator on institution letterhead. Orders will be billed at individual rate until proof of status is received. Foreign air speed delivery is included in all *Clinics* subscription prices. All prices are subject to change without notice. **POSTMASTER:** Send address changes to *Neurologic Clinics*, Elsevier Health Sciences Division, Subscription Customer Service, 3251 Riverport Lane, Maryland Heights, MO 63043. **Customer Service: Telephone: 1-800-654-2452 (U.S. and Canada); 314-447-8871 (outside U.S. and Canada). Fax: 314-447-8029. E-mail: journalscustomerservice-usa@elsevier.com (for print support); journalsonlinesupport-usa@elsevier.com (for online support).**

Reprints. For copies of 100 or more of articles in this publication, please contact the Commercial Reprints Department, Elsevier Inc., 360 Park Avenue South, New York, New York, 10010-1710; Tel.: +1-212-633-3874; Fax: +1-212-633-3820, and E-mail: reprints@elsevier.com.

Neurologic Clinics is also published in Spanish by Nueva Editorial Interamericana S.A., Mexico City, Mexico.

Neurologic Clinics is covered in *Current Contents/Clinical Medicine, MEDLINE/PubMed (Index Medicus), EMBASE/Excerpta Medica, and PsycINFO, and ISI/BIOMED.*

Contributors

CONSULTING EDITOR

RANDOLPH W. EVANS, MD
Clinical Professor, Department of Neurology, Baylor College of Medicine, Houston, Texas, USA

EDITORS

MAZEN M. DIMACHKIE, MD, FAAN, FANA
Professor & Director, Neuromuscular Division, Executive Vice Chairman & Vice Chairman for Research Programs Department of Neurology, Associate Director, Institute for Neurological Discoveries, University of Kansas Medical Center, Kansas City, Kansas, USA

RICHARD J. BAROHN, MD
Gertrude and Dewey Ziegler Professor of Neurology, University Distinguished Professor, Vice Chancellor for Research, President of the Research Institute Director, Frontiers: University of Kansas Clinical & Translational Science Institute, University of Kansas Medical Center, Kansas City, Kansas, USA

AUTHORS

MOHAMMED AL-HAIDAR, MD
Visiting Scholar, Department of Neurology, The George Washington University, Washington, DC, USA

CAROLINA BARNETT, MD, PhD
Assistant Professor, Neurology (Medicine), University of Toronto, University Health Network, Toronto, Ontario, Canada

RICHARD J. BAROHN, MD
Gertrude and Dewey Ziegler Professor of Neurology, University Distinguished Professor, Vice Chancellor for Research, President of the Research Institute Director, Frontiers: University of Kansas Clinical & Translational Science Institute, University of Kansas Medical Center, Kansas City, Kansas, USA

MICHAEL BENATAR, MD, PhD
Professor of Neurology, Department of Neurology, University of Miami, Miami, Florida, USA

EMMA CIAFALONI, MD
Professor of Neurology and Pediatrics, Director of Pediatric Neuromuscular Medicine, Department of Neurology, Neuromuscular Division, University of Rochester Medical Center, Rochester, New York, USA

MAZEN M. DIMACHKIE, MD, FAAN, FANA
Professor & Director, Neuromuscular Division, Executive Vice Chairman & Vice
Chairman for Research Programs Department of Neurology, Associate Director,
Institute for Neurological Discoveries, University of Kansas Medical Center,
Kansas City, Kansas, USA

CONSTANTINE FARMAKIDIS, MD
Assistant Professor, University of Kansas Medical Center, Kansas City, Kansas, USA

JOHANNA HAMEL, MD
Senior Instructor, Department of Neurology, Neuromuscular Division, University of
Rochester Medical Center, Rochester, New York, USA

MICHAEL K. HEHIR, MD
Associate Professor, Department of Neurosciences, The Robert Larner, M.D. College of
Medicine, University of Vermont, Burlington, Vermont, USA

LAURA HERBELIN, BSc, CCRP
Clinical Research Instructor of Neurology, University of Kansas Medical Center, Kansas
City, Kansas, USA

HENRY J. KAMINSKI, MD
Professor of Neurology, Department of Neurology, The George Washington University,
Washington, DC, USA

VITA G. KESNER, MD, PhD
Associate Professor of Neurology, Emory University School of Medicine, Atlanta, Georgia,
USA

ROBERT P. LISAK, MD, FRCP, FAAN, FANA
Parker Webber Chair in Neurology, Professor of Neurology, and Biochemistry,
Microbiology and Immunology, Wayne State University School of Medicine, Detroit
Medical Center, Detroit, Michigan, USA

LIN MEI, PhD
Professor and Chairman, Department of Neuroscience and Regenerative Medicine,
Augusta University, Augusta, Georgia, USA

HIROSHI NISHIMUNE, PhD
Associate Professor, Department of Anatomy and Cell Biology, University of Kansas
School of Medicine, Kansas City, Kansas, USA

SHIN J. OH, MD
Distinguished Professor Emeritus, Department of Neurology, University of Alabama at
Birmingham, Birmingham, Alabama, USA

MAMATHA PASNOOR, MD
Associate Professor of Neurology, Program Director, Clinical Neurophysiology,
Associate Program Director, Neurology Residency Program, Associate Program Director
for Neurophysiology and Neuromuscular Medicine, University of Kansas Medical Center,
Kansas City, Kansas, USA

MICHAEL H. RIVNER, MD
Professor of Neurology, EMG Lab, Augusta University, Augusta, Georgia, USA

ROBERT L. RUFF, MD, PhD
Professor Emeritus of Neurology and Neurosciences, Case Western University School of Medicine, The Metro Health System, Case Western Reserve University, Cleveland, Ohio, USA

PERRY B. SHIEH, MD, PhD
Associate Professor, Department of Neurology, University of California, Los Angeles, Los Angeles, California, USA

KAZUHIRO SHIGEMOTO, MD, PhD
Team Leader, Research Team for Geriatric Medicine, Tokyo Metropolitan Institute of Gerontology, Tokyo, Japan

NICHOLAS J. SILVESTRI, MD
Associate Professor, Department of Neurology, Jacobs School of Medicine and Biomedical Sciences, University at Buffalo, The State University of New York, Buffalo, New York, USA

Contents

> Neuromuscular junctions (NMJs) form between nerve terminals of spinal cord motor neurons and skeletal muscles, and perisynaptic Schwann cells and kranocytes cap NMJs. One muscle fiber has one NMJ, which is innervated by one motor nerve terminal. NMJs are excitatory synapses that use P/Q-type voltage-gated calcium channels to release the neurotransmitter acetylcholine. Acetylcholine receptors accumulate at the postsynaptic specialization called the end plate on the muscle fiber membrane, the sarcolemma. Proteins essential for the organization of end plates include agrin secreted from nerve terminals, Lrp4 and MuSK receptors for agrin, and Dok-7 and rapsyn cytosolic proteins in the muscle.

> Ocular myasthenia is a form of myasthenia gravis in which weakness is restricted to the ocular muscles and may produce significant visual disability. Patients present with fluctuating ptosis, diplopia, or a combination of both. Examination may show any type of ocular motility deficit ranging from isolated muscle palsy to complete ophthalmoplegia. Cogan lid twitch, enhanced ptosis, peek sign, and saccadic fatigue are specific examination findings that support the clinical diagnosis of myasthenia gravis. Confirmation of the diagnosis is challenging with autoantibody serology, and repetitive nerve stimulation studies are often negative.

> Myasthenia gravis (MG) is a rare disease but the most common disorder of the neuromuscular junction. It is the prototypic autoimmune disease most commonly caused by antibodies to the acetylcholine receptor (AChR) leading to characteristic fatigable weakness of the ocular, bulbar, respiratory, axial, and limb muscles. The majority of patients with MG first present with ocular symptoms. Most patients with MG experience at least 1 exacerbation of symptoms throughout the course of their illness. This article covers the epidemiology, clinical presentation, classification, and natural history of MG.

> Myasthenia gravis (MG) diagnosis is primarily clinically based. By the end
> of the clinical evaluation, clinicians have a sense as to whether presenting
> symptoms and elicited signs are weakly or strongly supportive of MG.
> Diagnostic tests can reaffirm the clinicians' impression. Edrophonium
> testing is rarely used but helpful in cases of measurable ptosis. Decre-
> mental response on slow-frequency repetitive nerve stimulation has a
> modest diagnostic yield in ocular MG but is helpful in generalized MG
> cases. The most sensitive test is single-fiber electromyography. In this
> article, the authors review the diagnostic testing approach of practicing cli-
> nicians for suspected MG cases.

> This article discusses antibodies associated with immune-mediated myas-
> thenia gravis and the pathologic action of these antibodies at the neuro-
> muscular junctions of skeletal muscle. To explain how these antibodies
> act, we consider the physiology of neuromuscular transmission with
> emphasis on 4 features: the structure of the neuromuscular junction; the
> roles of postsynaptic acetylcholine receptors and voltage-gated Na^+
> channels in converting the chemical signal from the nerve terminal into a
> propagated action potential on the muscle fiber that triggers muscle
> contraction; the safety factor for neuromuscular transmission; and how
> the safety factor is reduced in different forms of autoimmune myasthenia
> gravis.

> Around 20% of patients with myasthenia gravis are acetylcholine receptor
> antibody negative; muscle-specific tyrosine kinase antibodies (MuSK)
> were identified as the cause of myasthenia gravis in 30% to 40% of these
> cases. Anti-MuSK myasthenia gravis is associated with specific clinical
> phenotypes. One is a bulbar form with fewer ocular symptoms. Others
> show an isolated head drop or symptoms indistinguishable from acetyl-
> choline receptor-positive myasthenia gravis. These patients usually
> respond well to immunosuppressive therapy but not as well to choli-
> nesterase inhibitors. Other antibodies associated with myasthenia
> gravis, including low-density lipoprotein receptor-related protein 4, are
> discussed.

> With specialized care, patients with myasthenia gravis can have very
> good outcomes. The mainstays of treatment are acetylcholinesterase

inhibitors and immunosuppressive and immunomodulatory therapies. There is good evidence that thymectomy is beneficial in thymomatous and nonthymomatous disease. Nearly all of the drugs used for MG are considered "off-label." The 2 exceptions are acetylcholinesterase inhibitors and complement inhibition with eculizumab, which was recently approved by the US Food and Drug Administration for myasthenia gravis. This article reviews the evidence base and provides a framework for the treatment of myasthenia gravis, highlighting recent additions to the literature.

This article provides an overview of health-related outcome measurement to better understand what different outcomes used in myasthenia actually measure and to provide some guidance when choosing measures based on the clinical context and question. In myasthenia, the most commonly used outcome measures are aimed at assessing the signs and symptoms. The authors provide a summary of the most commonly used outcome measures. They discuss instruments that gauge disease overall health impact, such as on disability and quality of life. Finally, they discuss other relevant outcomes such as steroid-sparing effects and the role of surrogate markers.

Myasthenia gravis presents a risk factor for pregnancy and delivery and can affect the birth process and the newborn. In return, pregnancy can affect the course of myasthenia and worsen the disease during pregnancy, requiring treatment modifications. Treatment optimization and drug safety should be addressed before conception. Delivery is complicated by prolonged labor. Newborns can develop neonatal myasthenia gravis, a treatable and transient disease. Patients should not be discouraged to become pregnant but be provided with supportive counseling, planning, and monitoring in a multidisciplinary team involving obstetrician, anesthesiologist, pediatrician, and neurologist. Pregnancy outcome is favorable in women who receive treatment and expert care.

The congenital myasthenic syndromes (CMSs) are a group of rare genetic conditions characterized by abnormal neuromuscular transmission. Typically, these conditions have been the result of a dysfunctional protein that is present in the presynaptic terminal, the synaptic cleft, or the postsynaptic terminal. Many of these syndromes present within the first few years of life with fluctuating and fatigable weakness in a distribution similar to that of myasthenia gravis, although a limb-girdle distribution and late onset are also seen in certain specific types of CMS. Electrodiagnostic testing with repetitive nerve stimulation may be helpful in some forms of CMS.

Lambert-Eaton myasthenic syndrome is a paraneoplastic or primary
autoimmune neuromuscular junction disorder characterized by proximal
weakness, autonomic dysfunction and ariflexia. The characteristic symptoms are thought to be caused by antibodies generated against the
P/Q-type voltage-gated calcium channels present on presynaptic nerve
terminals and by diminished release of acetylcholine. More than half of
Lambert-Eaton myasthenic syndrome cases are associated with small
cell lung carcinoma. Diagnosis is confirmed by serologic testing and electrophysiologic studies. 3,4-diaminopyridine is effective symptomatic treatment of LEMS.

NEUROLOGIC CLINICS

THE CLINICS ARE AVAILABLE ONLINE!
Access your subscription at:
www.theclinics.com

NEUROLOGIC CLINICS

FORTHCOMING ISSUES

August 2018
Neuro-oncology
Patrick Y. Wen and Eudocia Q. Lee, Editors

November 2018
Neuro-infectious Diseases
Russell E. Bartt and Allen J. Aksamit, Jr, Editors

February 2019
Neurology of Pregnancy
Mary Angela O'Neal, Editor

RECENT ISSUES

February 2017
Multiple Sclerosis
Darin T. Okuda, Editor

November 2017
Neurocritical Care
Alejandro A. Rabinstein, Editor

August 2017
Sports Neurology
Tad Seifert, Editor

RELATED INTEREST

Neuroimaging Clinics of North America, January 2018 (Vol. 28, Issue 1)
Cerebral Microbleeds
Michael G. Fehlings, Editor

THE CLINICS ARE AVAILABLE ONLINE!
Access your subscription at:
www.theclinics.com

Preface

Fifty Key Publications on Myasthenia Gravis and Related Disorders

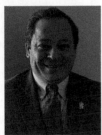 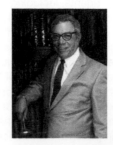

Mazen M. Dimachkie, MD, FAAN, FANA   Richard J. Barohn, MD
Editors

We are once again delighted to guest edit an issue of *Neurologic Clinics* on a neuromuscular topic. Previously, we cowrote and edited issues on peripheral neuropathy, myopathy, and motor neuron disease. The current issue is focused on disorders of the neuromuscular junction (NMJ), predominantly myasthenia gravis (MG), but also with information on Lambert-Eaton myasthenic syndrome (LFMS) and congenital myasthenic syndromes. In this preface, we want to briefly provide an overview of the history of MG. We have provided references that we consider some of the fifty most important publications on MG and related disorders.

MG was suspected as a disease probably since Thomas Willis first wrote about "the palsy" in the late 1600s.[1] In the late 1800s, MG was defined as a clinical entity by German neurologists; Wilhelm Erb, Samuel Goldflam, Herman Oppenheim, and Friedrich Jolly described the decremental muscle response on electrophysiologic testing.[2–5] The modern era that marks our understanding of MG can be dated to the first half of the twentieth century. In this time period, the two discoveries that led to a better understanding of MG involved the thymus gland's relation to MG and the drug treatment for MG. Thymoma and enlarged thymus glands were observed on autopsy in MG patients.[6–8] Sauerbach first successfully removed an enlarged thymus gland in 1911.[9] In the 1930s and 1940s, Blalock and colleagues[10,11] became leaders advocating thymectomy for MG patients with and without thymoma. Over the next 50 years, the belief that thymectomy was beneficial for MG grew, and this became standard of care despite the lack of an adequately controlled trial.[12] The second major discovery in the first half of the twentieth century was the finding that the use of acetylcholinesterase inhibitors would improve the symptoms and signs of MG. Mary Walker in England was the first to observe such improvement with the drugs physostigmine[13] and neostigmine.[14] Twenty years later, pyridostigmine bromide was introduced, and this drug remains a mainstay in our treatment of MG.[15,16]

Neurol Clin 36 (2018) xiii–xvii
https://doi.org/10.1016/j.ncl.2018.03.001
0733-8619/18/© 2018 Published by Elsevier Inc.

neurologic.theclinics.com

The next significant breakthroughs in the field occurred in the second half of the twentieth century when a number of discoveries occurred: (1) an understanding of the neuroanatomy and neurochemistry of the NMJ[17]; (2) development of the animal model of experimental allergic MG[18]; (3) the discovery of antibodies to the acetylcholine receptor (AChR) in humans with MG and passive transfer of MG to mice from human immunoglobulin of MG patients[19–21]; (4) passive transfer of MG to mice from human immunoglobulin of MG patients[22]; (5) the discovery that corticosteroids and other immunosuppressive agents, including plasmapheresis, can improve MG symptoms and signs; and finally,[23–31] (6) the development of mechanical ventilation to keep patients alive when they go into respiratory failure from myasthenia crisis. During this era, the electrophysiologic techniques for diagnosing MG improved as did the equipment so that it became expected for medical practitioners to be able to assess NMJ physiology routinely in patients suspected of MG. In addition to repetitive nerve stimulation, the technique of single-fiber electromyography was introduced by Stalberg and was shown to be extremely sensitive for detecting NMJ abnormalities that supported the clinical diagnosis of MG.[32] In the 1950s, the disorder known as LEMS was described, initially in patients with cancer and later in noncancer patients.[33] In the 1970s, the first congenital myasthenic syndrome was described.[34]

Now we are entering a new era of innovation in the field. First, new autoantibodies are being discovered that are responsible for NMJ disorders. The first of these was antibodies to voltage-gated P-/Q-type calcium channels in LEMS.[35] This was followed by the discovery of MuSK antibodies in some patients with MG, and more recently, other antibodies have been identified, including those to LRP4, rapsyn, agrin, and more recently, cortactin.[36,37] Antibodies to MuSK and LRP4 are now commercially available so the percent of true antibody-negative patients with generalized MG is lower than it used to be 20 years ago. Second, we now have a great deal of experience in clinical research in MG and have refined the endpoint measurements and trial designs. A new classification system for MG and new standards for MG clinical trials were published by a committee of the Myasthenia Gravis Foundation of America[38] and new measures continue to be described. Our group refined the quantitative MG scale and developed the MG Activity of Daily Living scale.[39,40] Subsequently, Ted Burns and colleagues designed the useful MG composite scale incorporating the best aspects of prior measures.[41] Other measures continue to be developed by the next generation of MG researchers, such as Carolina Barnett-Tapia, who developed the MG impairment index with colleagues in Toronto.[42]

In this new era, we have seen advances in immune suppression and immunomodulating therapy for MG. With the completion and publication of the landmark thymectomy trial in MG, we can now say with conviction that patients with MG who undergo thymectomy improve and their prednisone dose can be lowered more than patients who do not have a thymectomy.[43] The article by Dr Gil Wolfe and colleagues published in the New England Journal of Medicine in 2016 is a landmark in the field of neuromuscular medicine. In addition, novel therapies are being developed for MG through rigorous clinical trials. Prior to 2000, we could find only seven randomized controlled published MG trials. As of 2018, 22 randomized clinical trials have been published for MG. Recently, this led to the US Food and Drug Administration approval of the complement inhibitor eculizumab (Soliris®) for adult patients with generalized MG who are AChR antibody positive. In phase 2 and 3 studies, this drug significantly improved MG patients.[44,45] This drug and other drugs that are being developed in this class have the potential of transforming the treatment of this disease. This recent finding was built on early findings demonstrating increased complement in the serum of MG patients and the presence of complements at the NMJ in MG.[46,47] We have learned a great deal from recent clinical trials that have yielded negative results.[48–50] Other pharmaceutical companies are trying equally novel approaches to treat MG, and many trials are in progress. MG indeed used to be a grave disease with 30% mortality. Now, with the advent of all the advances and others described above, everyone we see with MG should improve, and it should be a rare event indeed for a patient to die of MG.

We had anticipated a contribution to this issue by our dear friend and colleague, Dr Claudio Mazia, who unfortunately died before he could add his MG expertise to this important publication. We would like to thank all of the authors of these articles in this issue for their expertise in the field and for spending the time to put their knowledge in this format so it can be shared with others.

Mazen M. Dimachkie, MD, FAAN, FANA
Professor & Director, Neuromuscular Division
Executive Vice Chairman & Vice Chairman for
Research Programs Department of Neurology
Associate Director, Institute for Neurological Discoveries
University of Kansas Medical Center
3901 Rainbow Boulevard, Mail Stop 2012
Kansas City, KS 66160, USA

Richard J. Barohn, MD
Gertrude and Dewey Ziegler Professor of Neurology
University Distinguished Professor
Vice Chancellor for Research
President of the Research Institute
Director, Frontiers: University of Kansas Clinical
& Translational Science Institute
University of Kansas Medical Center
3901 Rainbow Boulevard, Mail Stop 2012
Kansas City, KS 66160, USA

E-mail addresses:
mdimachkie@kumc.edu (M.M. Dimachkie)
rbarohn@kumc.edu (R.J. Barohn)

REFERENCES

1. Willis T. The London practice of physick, or the whole practical part of the physick contained in the works of Dr Willis. London: Adams LB; 1685. p. 431–2. The Classics of Neurology and Neurosurgery. New York: 1991 [reprint].

2. Erb W. Sur Casiusitik der bulbären Lähmungen. Arch Psychiatr Nervenkr (1970) 1879;9:336–50 [in German].

3. Goldflam S. Ueber einen scheinbar heilbaren bulbärparlytischen Symptomencomplext mit Betheiligung der Extremitäten. Deitsche Zeitchrift für Nervenheilkndle 1893;4:312–52 [in German].

4. Oppenheim H. Die Myastenische Paralyse (Bulbarparalyse ohne anatomischen Befund). Berlin: JHH Karger; 1901 [in German].

5. Jolly Fl. Ueber Myasthenia gravis pseudoparalytica. Berliner Klinische Wochenschrift 1895;32:1–7 [in German].

6. Wiegert C. Pathologisch-anatomischer Beitrag zur Erb'schen Krankheit (Myasthenia gravis). Neurol Zentralblatt 1901;20:597–601 [in German].

7. Bell ET. Tumors of the thymus in myasthenia gravis. J Nerv Ment Dis 1917;45:130–43.

8. Norris EH. The thymoma and thymic hyperplasia in myasthenia gravis with observations on the general pathology. Am J Cancer 1936;27:421–33.
9. Schumacher CH, Roth P. Thymektomie bei einem Fall von Murbus Basedowi mit Myastenia. Mittelungren aus den Grenzgebeiten der Medizin und Chirurrgi 1913; 25:746–65.
10. Blalock A, Mason MF, Morgan HJ, et al. Myasthenia gravis and tumors of the thymic region: report of a case in which the tumor was removed. Ann Surg 1939;110:544–59.
11. Blalock A, Harvey AM, Ford FF, et al. The treatment of myasthenia gravis by removal of the thymus gland. J Am Med Assoc 1941;117:1529–33.
12. Gronseth GS, Barohn RJ. Practice parameter: thymectomy for autoimmune myasthenia gravis (an evidence-based review): report of the Quality Standards Subcommittee of the American Academy of Neurology. Neurology 2000;55(1):7–15.
13. Walker MB. Treatment of myasthenia gravis with physostigmine. Lancet 1934;1: 1200–1.
14. Walker M. Case showing the effect of prostigmin on myasthenia gravis. Proc R Soc Med 1935;28:759–61.
15. Osserman KE, Teng P, Kaplan LI. Studies in myasthenia gravis; preliminary report on therapy with mestinon bromide. J Am Med Assoc 1954;155(11):961–5.
16. Schwab RS, Timberlake WH. Pyridostigmin (mestinon) in the treatment of myasthenia gravis. N Engl J Med 1954;251(7):271–2.
17. Santa T, Engel AG, Lambert EH. Histometric study of neuromuscular junction ultrastructure I. Myasthenia gravis. Neurology 1972;22:71–82.
18. Patrick J, Lindstrom J. Autoimmune response to acetylcholine receptor. Science 1973;180:871–2.
19. Appel SH, Almon RR, Levy N. Acetylcholine receptor antibodies in myasthenia gravis. N Engl J Med 1975;293:760–1.
20. Lindstrom JM, Seybold ME, Lennon VA, et al. Antibody to acetylcholine receptor in myasthenia gravis. Neurology 1976;26:1054–9.
21. Bender AN, Engel WK, Ringel SP, et al. Myasthenia gravis: a serum factor blocking acetylcholine receptors of the human neuromuscular junction. Lancet 1975;1:607–9.
22. Tokya KV, Drachman DB, Griffith DE, et al. Study of humoral immune mechanisms by passive transfer to mice. N Engl J Med 1977;296:125–30.
23. Warmolts JR, Engel WK. Benefit from alternate-day prednisone in myasthenia gravis. N Engl J Med 1972;286:17–20.
24. Jenkins RB. Treatment of myasthenia gravis with prednisone. Lancet 1972; 1(7754):765–7.
25. Pazcuzi RM, Coslett HB, Johns TR. Long-term corticosteroid treatment of myasthenia gravis: report of 116 patients. Ann Neurol 1984;15(3):291–8.
26. Pinching AJ, Peters DK. Remission of myasthenia gravis following plasma-exchange. Lancet 1976;2(8000):1373–6.
27. Dau PC, Lindstrom JM, Cassel CK, et al. Plasmapheresis and immunosuppressive drug therapy in myasthenia gravis. N Engl J Med 1977;297(21):1134–40.
28. Tindall RS, Rollins JA, Phillips JT, et al. Preliminary results of a double-blind, randomized, placebo-controlled trial of cyclosporine in myasthenia gravis. N Engl J Med 1987;316(12):719–24.
29. Tindall RS, Phillips JT, Rollins JA, et al. A clinical therapeutic trial of cyclosporine in myasthenia gravis. Ann N Y Acad Sci 1993;681:539–51.
30. Palace J, Newsom-Davis J, Lecky B. A randomized double-blind trial of prednisolone alone or with azathioprine in myasthenia gravis. Myasthenia Gravis Study Group. Neurology 1998;50(6):1778–83.

31. Zinman L, Ng E, Bril V. IV immunoglobulin in patients with myasthenia gravis: a randomized controlled trial. Neurology 2007;68(11):837–41.
32. Ekstedt J, Stålberg E. The effect of non-paralytic doses of D-tubocurarine on individual motor end-plates in man, studied with a new electrophysiological method. Electroencephalogr Clin Neurophysiol 1969;27(6):557–62.
33. Lambert EH, Eaton LM, Rooke ED. Defect of neuromuscular conduction associated with malignant neoplasms. Am J Physiol 1956;187:612–3.
34. Engel AG, Lambert EH, Gomez MR. A new myasthenic syndrome with end-plate acetylcholinesterase deficiency, small nerve terminals, and reduced acetylcholine release. Ann Neurol 1977;1(4):315–30.
35. Lennon VA, Lambert EH. Antibodies bind solubilized calcium channel-omega-conotoxin complexes from small cell lung carcinoma: a diagnostic aid for Lambert-Eaton myasthenic syndrome. Mayo Clin Proc 1989;64:1498.
36. Hoch W, McConville J, Helms S, et al. Auto-antibodies to the receptor tyrosine kinase MuSK in patients with myasthenia gravis without acetylcholine receptor antibodies. Nat Med 2001;7:365–8.
37. Zhang B, Tzartos JS, Belimezi M, et al. Autoantibodies to lipoprotein-related protein 4 in patients with double-seronegative myasthenia gravis. Arch Neurol 2012;69:445–51.
38. Jaretzki A 3rd, Barohn RJ, Ernstoff RM, et al. Myasthenia gravis: recommendations for clinical research standards. Task Force of the Medical Scientific Advisory Board of the Myasthenia Gravis Foundation of America. Neurology 2000;55(1):16–23.
39. Barohn RJ, McIntire D, Herbelin L, et al. Reliability testing of the quantitative myasthenia gravis score. Ann N Y Acad Sci 1998;841:769–72.
40. Wolfe GI, Herbelin L, Nations SP, et al. Myasthenia gravis activities of daily living profile. Neurology 1999;52:1487–9.
41. Burns TB, Conaway MR, Cutter GR, et al. The Muscle Study Group. Less is more, or almost as much: a 15-item quality-of-life instrument for myasthenia gravis. Muscle Nerve 2008;38(2):957–63.
42. Barnett C, Bril V, Kapral M, et al. Development and validation of the myasthenia gravis impairment index. Neurology 2016;87(9):879–86.
43. Wolfe GI, Kaminski HJ, Aban IB, et al. Randomized trial of thymectomy in myasthenia gravis. N Engl J Med 2016;375(6):511–22.
44. Howard JF Jr, Barohn RJ, Cutter GR, et al. A randomized, double-blind, placebo-controlled phase II study of eculizumab in patients with refractory generalized myasthenia gravis. Muscle Nerve 2013;48(1):76–84.
45. Howard JF Jr, Utsugisawa K, Benatar M, et al, REGAIN Study Group. Safety and efficacy of eculizumab in anti-acetylcholine receptor antibody-positive refractory generalised myasthenia gravis (REGAIN): a phase 3, randomised, double-blind, placebo-controlled, multicentre study. Lancet Neurol 2017;16(12):976–86.
46. Nastuk WL, Plescia OJ, Osserman KE. Changes in serum complement activity in patients with myasthenia gravis. Proc Soc Exp Biol Med 1960;105:177–84.
47. Engel AG, Lambert EH, Howard FM. Immune complexes (IgG and C3) at the motor end-plate in myasthenia gravis: ultrastructural and light microscopic localization and electrophysiologic correlations. Mayo Clin Proc 1977;52:627.
48. Muscle Study Group. A trial of mycophenolate mofetil with prednisone as initial immunotherapy myasthenia gravis. Neurology 2008;71(6):394–9.
49. Sanders DB, Hart IK, Mantegazza R, et al. An international, phase III, randomized trial of mycophenolate mofetil in myasthenia gravis. Neurology 2008;71(6):400–6.
50. Pasnoor M, He J, Herbelin L, et al. A randomized controlled trial of methotrexate for patients with generalized myasthenia gravis. Neurology 2016;87(1):57–64.

Practical Anatomy of the Neuromuscular Junction in Health and Disease

Hiroshi Nishimune, PhD[a],*, Kazuhiro Shigemoto, MD, PhD[b]

KEYWORDS

- Neuromuscular junction • Motor neuron • Muscle • Active zone
- Acetylcholine receptors • MuSK • Voltage-gated calcium channels

KEY POINTS

- Neuromuscular junctions are excitatory chemical synapses that use acetylcholine as the neurotransmitter.
- Neuromuscular junctions form between nerve terminals of spinal cord motor neurons and skeletal muscles and are covered by perisynaptic Schwann cells and kranocytes.
- MuSK is indispensable for the accumulation of acetylcholine receptors at end plates.

NEUROMUSCULAR JUNCTIONS AND MOTOR NERVES

Neuromuscular junctions (NMJs) are excitatory chemical synapses formed between nerve terminals of spinal cord motor neurons and skeletal muscle fibers that use acetylcholine as the neurotransmitter. Muscle fibers in the skeletal muscles receive monosynaptic input directly from the lower motor neurons in the spinal cord (**Fig. 1**A). Therefore, motor neuron axons originating from the spinal cord travel a long distance to innervate muscle fibers. In most skeletal muscles, one muscle fiber has one NMJ. A mature NMJ is innervated by one motor nerve terminal (**Fig. 2**, *normal*); therefore, there is a one-to-one relationship between a given muscle fiber and motor neuron. However, one motor neuron innervates multiple muscle fibers by branching its axon within the innervation target muscle. This group of muscle fibers

Disclosure Statement: The authors have nothing to disclose.
This work was supported by grants from NIH USA, 1R01NS078214 and 1R01AG051470 (H. Nishimune), from MEXT Japan, Grant-in-Aid for Scientific Research B 24390228, and Challenging Exploratory Research 25670437 (K. Shigemoto).
[a] Department of Anatomy and Cell Biology, University of Kansas School of Medicine, 3901 Rainbow Boulevard, MS 3051, Hemenway Room 2073, Kansas City, KS 66160, USA;
[b] Research Team for Geriatric Medicine, Tokyo Metropolitan Institute of Gerontology, Sakae-cho 35-2, Itabashi-ku, Tokyo 173-0015, Japan
* Corresponding author.
E-mail address: hnishimune@kumc.edu

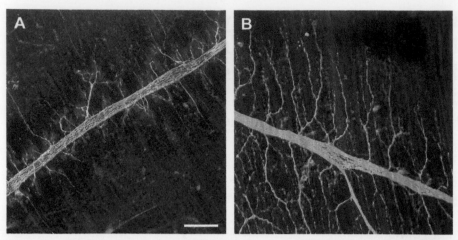

Fig. 1. Aberrant structures of presynaptic and postsynaptic differentiation in the diaphragm muscle from a MuSK$^{-/-}$ mutant mouse. A whole-mount diaphragm muscle from a wild-type (A) or a MuSK$^{-/-}$ mutant (B) was simultaneously stained with antibodies against neurofilament to label motor axons (green) and with rhodamine-labeled α-bungarotoxin to label acetylcholine receptors (red) on the postsynaptic muscle membrane. NMJs are not formed in MuSK$^{-/-}$ mutant mouse. Scale bar, 200 μm. (From Shigemoto K, Kubo S, Mori S, et al. The immunopathogenesis of experimental autoimmune myasthenia gravis induced by autoantibodies against muscle-specific kinase. In: Christadoss P, editor. Myasthenia gravis disease mechanisms and immune intervention. [Chapter 17]. New York: Linus Publication, Inc; 2009. p. 317; with permission.)

innervated by one motor neuron is called a motor unit. A nerve terminal innervates one NMJ and does not extend beyond the NMJ to innervate another muscle fiber (see **Fig. 2**, *normal*). This type of innervation differs from synapses of the central nervous system where axons can make *en passant* synapses or boutons *en passant* to form multiple synapses by one branch on an axon.

In the human diaphragm, two phrenic nerve bundles reach the center area of the right and left hemi-diaphragm. Each nerve bundle trifurcates and further splits in a radial fashion in the hemi-diaphragm, forming a net of nerve branches covering the muscle.[1] NMJs are often located in the center area of the muscle fibers and are arranged in a line among the nearby muscle fibers. The postsynaptic specialization of NMJs is often called the "end plate," also known as motor point, and the narrow distribution pattern of NMJs in a muscle is referred to as the "end plate band" (see **Fig. 1**A).

END PLATES AND ACETYLCHOLINE RECEPTORS

NMJs form in an indented area or a trough on the muscle cell membrane known as the synaptic gutter (primary gutter). These synaptic gutters are shown as a trough in scanning electron micrographs and an NMJ profile in transmission electron micrographs (**Fig. 3**, *control*). The postsynaptic muscle plasma membrane further invaginates to form the junctional folds (see **Fig. 3**B, *arrowhead*). These junctional folds extend from the postsynaptic membrane perpendicularly into the muscle cytosol. These junctional folds contribute to the increase in the muscle surface area to hold more acetylcholine receptors (AChRs) at the top of the junctional folds and part way down on the sides[2]; and the concentration of voltage-gated sodium channels at the trough of the

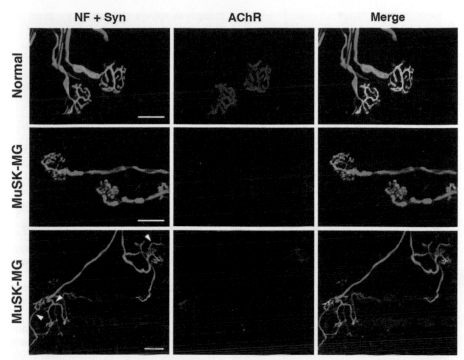

Fig. 2. Disorganization of presynaptic and postsynaptic structures of NMJs in MuSK-MG mice. Axons and nerve terminals (*green*) were stained with antineurofilament and antisynaptophysin antibodies (NF + Syn), and AChRs (*red*) were labeled with rhodamine-labeled α-bungarotoxin. Some NMJs with axon sprouts were observed in MuSK-MG mice (*arrowheads*). Scale bars: 30 μm. AChR, acetylcholine receptor; MG, myasthenia gravis. (*Reprinted from* Mori S, Kubo S, Akiyoshi T, et al. Antibodies against muscle-specific kinase impair both presynaptic and postsynaptic functions in a murine model of myasthenia gravis. Am J Pathol 2012;180(2):803; with permission from Elsevier Inc.)

junctional folds for generating action potentials in muscle fibers.[3] The synaptic gutter and junctional folds compose the end plates.

AChRs are ligand-gated cation channels. Their density is more than 1000-fold higher at the postsynaptic specialization than in extrasynaptic area of the muscle fiber cell membrane.[2,4] AChR subunits assemble a functional pentamer as $\alpha_2\beta\gamma\delta$ and insert into the cell membrane.[2,5] Acetylcholine binds to the extracellular domain of the α subunits on opposite sides of the channel pore.[6] The half-life of AChR is approximately 14 days at NMJs of living adult mice.[7] In patients with myasthenia gravis (MG), IgG1 autoantibodies against the AChR α1-subunit cause progressive degeneration of the junctional folds and widening of the synaptic cleft.[8]

SYNAPTIC CLEFT

Motor nerve terminals fill the synaptic gutter to form NMJs. However, motor nerve terminals and muscle fibers do not make direct contact or form a cell adhesion complex, which is one the differences between NMJs and synapses of the central nervous system. Cell membranes of motor nerve terminals and muscle fibers are separated by a space called the synaptic cleft, which is approximately 30 to 50 nm. In the synaptic

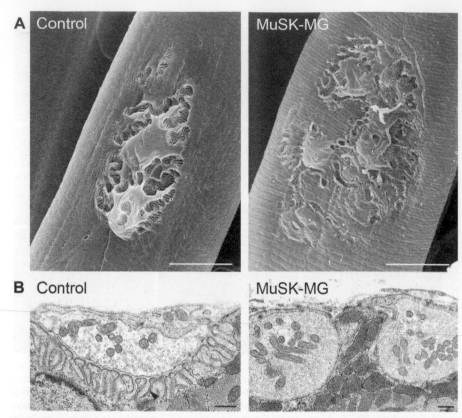

Fig. 3. Disruption of the NMJ ultrastructure in MuSK-MG mice. (*A*) Complex synaptic gutters containing numerous slitlike junctional folds (control) were observed at NMJs of control tibialis anterior muscle by scanning electron microscopy. Synaptic gutter flattening and fewer slitlike junctional folds were observed in NMJs of MuSK-MG mice (MuSK-MG). Scale bars: 15 mm. (*B*) Evenly distributed junctional folds (*arrowhead*) of comparable depth were observed in control animals via transmission electron microscopy. A loss of junctional folds was observed in MuSK-MG mice. Scale bars: 500 nm. (*Reprinted from* Mori S, Kubo S, Akiyoshi T, et al. Antibodies against muscle-specific kinase impair both presynaptic and postsynaptic functions in a murine model of myasthenia gravis. Am J Pathol 2012;180(2):803; with permission from Elsevier Inc.)

cleft, acetylcholinesterase is concentrated to hydrolyze the neurotransmitter acetylcholine to terminate each synaptic transmission. The synaptic cleft is filled with extracellular matrix forming the basal lamina.[9,10] The extrasynaptic area of the sarcolemma, the cell membrane of muscle fibers, is surrounded by the internal basal lamina layer and external reticular lamina layer that form the connective tissue layer also called the basement membrane.[9,10] The basal lamina consists of collagens, fibronectins, laminins, nidogens, and perlecan.[9–11] These extracellular matrix proteins form an interwoven matrix in the synaptic cleft. Furthermore, NMJ-specific extracellular matrix proteins have been identified, including collagen IV $\alpha2$, $\alpha3$, and $\alpha6$ chains; collagen XIII; and laminin $\alpha4$, $\alpha5$, and $\beta2$ chains.[12] These synaptic cleft–specific extracellular matrix proteins have functional roles for the organization and maintenance of the presynaptic and postsynaptic specialization of NMJs.[12–15]

PRESYNAPTIC TERMINALS

Mature NMJs show a branched and complex morphology (see **Fig. 2**, *normal*). A motor nerve terminal faithfully traces the distribution pattern of an AChR cluster. A nerve terminal of a normal/healthy NMJ occupies most of the region of an AChR cluster with a near complete overlap (see **Fig. 2**, *normal*, *merge*). At the ultrastructural level, using transmission electron microscopy analysis, three main structures are identified: active zones, mitochondria, and synaptic vesicles 30 to 50 nm in diameter (see **Fig. 3**B, *control*). Synaptic vesicles of NMJs contain the neurotransmitter acetylcholine and are localized near the presynaptic membrane. Specifically, synaptic vesicles accumulate at active zones of the presynaptic membrane.

The active zones are synaptic vesicle release sites where synaptic vesicles accumulate and fuse with the presynaptic membrane for exocytotic release of the neurotransmitter acetylcholine.[16,17] These active zones appear as electron-dense material protruding into the cytosolic side from the presynaptic membrane (motor neuron cell membrane) in electron micrographs (see **Fig. 3**B, *control*). These active zones are often found at the presynaptic membrane area facing the mouth of postsynaptic junctional folds, indicating an alignment of presynaptic and postsynaptic specialization. The active zones are composed of P/Q-type voltage-gated calcium channels and the cytoskeletal matrix at the active zone, which includes Bassoon, ELKS/CAST2/Erc1, Munc13, Piccolo, and Rab3-interacting proteins 1 and 2 (RIM1/2). Calcium channels trigger synaptic transmissions, and cytoskeletal matrix at the active zone proteins play roles in synaptic vesicle accumulation and functional modification of the calcium channels.[18,19] These P/Q-type voltage-gated calcium channels at NMJs are one of the targets for Lambert-Eaton myasthenia syndrome autoantibodies. The passive transfer mouse model of Lambert-Eaton myasthenia syndrome exhibits fewer active zones.[20] A similar decrease in active zone number was observed when the interaction between P/Q-type voltage-gated calcium channels and their extracellular ligand was perturbed, suggesting a role of active zones in the cause of Lambert-Eaton myasthenia syndrome in addition to the decreased function of P/Q-type voltage-gated calcium channels.[21]

When action potentials reach presynaptic terminals, voltage-gated calcium channels open and induce calcium influx at the active zones. The rise in the calcium concentration induces a conformational change of Soluble NSF Attachment Protein Receptor (SNARE) proteins (synaptobrevin/VAMP, SNAP-25, syntaxin 1) and the fusion of docked synaptic vesicles with the presynaptic membrane. Acetylcholine is then released by exocytosis, spreads by diffusion across the synaptic cleft, binds to AChRs concentrated at the postsynaptic membrane, and causes depolarization of the muscle fibers for contraction. Synaptic vesicle-related proteins involved in this process accumulate at presynaptic terminals, including the calcium sensor synaptotagmin and synaptophysin, synapsin I, and synaptic vesicle protein 2.

CELLS CAPPING NEUROMUSCULAR JUNCTIONS

NMJs are covered by glia cells called perisynaptic Schwann cells (also known as terminal Schwann cells, **Fig. 3**B, *control*).[22–24] These perisynaptic Schwann cells contribute to the maintenance of the NMJ structure, synaptic transmission efficiency, and the regeneration of NMJs.[22,25–27] Ablation of perisynaptic Schwann cells causes the degeneration of NMJs in experimental animal models.[25,26] In addition, a fourth cell type has been identified at the NMJs and has been named kranocytes.[28] The kranocytes cap NMJs above the perisynaptic Schwann cells and play roles in nerve regeneration and sprouting.[23,28]

MOLECULAR MECHANISM OF NEUROMUSCULAR JUNCTION ORGANIZATION

The molecular mechanisms of NMJ differentiation/organization have been studied actively, and the knowledge has contributed to the better understanding of MG. In short, proteoglycan agrin is secreted from nerve terminals and binds to postsynaptic receptors composed of low-density lipoprotein receptor–related protein 4 (LRP4) and MuSK (muscle-specific kinase).[29–33] This signaling induces cytosolic proteins Dok-7 and rapsyn to accumulate AChR and postsynaptic specialization.[34–37] In MG, transmembrane proteins, AChRs, and MuSK become targets of autoantibodies. The roles of MuSK are described in detail next.

MuSK IS INDISPENSABLE FOR THE DEVELOPMENT OF NEUROMUSCULAR JUNCTIONS

MuSK is a receptor-tyrosine kinase that is concentrated at the tips of synaptic folds in the NMJs along with AChRs.[38] MuSK is activated through an association with LRP4 and agrin, a nerve-derived heparan sulfate proteoglycan.[29,39–41] MuSK is also activated by its interaction with Dok-7, a cytoplasmic adaptor-like protein, without binding to agrin and Lrp4.[37,42] These dual activation mechanisms of MuSK are required for the formation of NMJs during the developing stages of an embryo.[29,37,39] MuSK knockout mice display devastating defects in both presynaptic and postsynaptic differentiation and die at birth because of apnea. In the mutant mice, branches of the main intramuscular nerve grow excessively and fail to establish normal contacts between specialized nerve terminals and the muscle, where AChR clusters are present on myotubes opposing ingrowing nerve terminals in the normal mouse (see **Fig. 1**).[29] Furthermore, the nerve fibers cannot stop and wander aimlessly across the muscle width.[29] MuSK activates the signaling cascades required for all aspects of NMJ formation, including postsynaptic organization and postsynaptic differentiation by regulating the elaboration of retrograde signals. The same structural defects have been demonstrated in Dok-7 knock-out mice.[37]

THE ROLES OF MuSK IN MATURE NEUROMUSCULAR JUNCTIONS

Is MuSK required for the maintenance of NMJs and during development? If so, what roles does MuSK play in mature NMJs? Important clues for the functions of MuSK in mature NMJs have been obtained by the study of pathogenic mechanisms of MuSK-MG. MuSK-MG patients often have severe bulbar dysfunction and respiratory insufficiency, and anti-MuSK antibodies in the patients predominantly belong to the IgG4 subclass, which does not activate the classical complement pathway.[43–52] The absence of destruction mechanisms against NMJs by the autoantibodies in MuSK-MG patients provided the evidence to understand the roles of MuSK in the maintenance of the function and structure of NMJs. As observed in the patients, severe generalized MG was caused by passive transfer of the human IgG4 subclass derived from MuSK-MG patients into mice or by active immunization of the recombinant MuSK protein into rabbits strain.[53,54] The pathologic changes in the NMJs of these animal models included a significant loss of AChR expression and a reduction in junctional folds at postsynaptic membranes (see **Figs. 2** and **3**).[55] These striking alterations indicated that MuSK is indispensable for the maintenance of postsynaptic structures at mature NMJs.

Intriguingly, the morphologic changes were not confined to the postsynaptic membrane where MuSK is selectively expressed. Reductions in the size of NMJs and a retraction of motor terminals from NMJs have been observed in patients and MuSK-MG animals (see **Fig. 3**).[53–57] In addition, electrophysiologic studies have

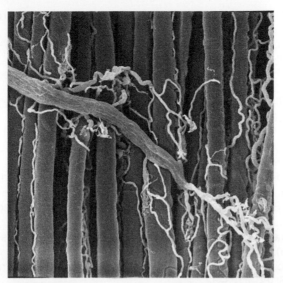

Fig. 4. Increased branching of intramuscular nerve fibers was observed in MuSK-MG mice by scanning electron microscopy.

demonstrated functional defects in postsynaptic AChRs and presynaptic terminals. Acetylcholine sensitivity was reduced as a result of the loss of postsynaptic AChRs; however, a compensatory increase in acetylcholine release from presynaptic terminals was also lacking in MuSK-MG patients and animal models.[55,57] 3,4-Diaminopyridine, a drug that increases the release of acetylcholine quanta, can alleviate the impairment in the compensatory responses In MuSK-MG patients and animals.[58–60] In contrast, compensatory acetylcholine release from presynaptic terminals is preserved as a homeostatic response in AChR-MG patients and animals.[56,57] Because MuSK is selectively expressed in skeletal muscle but not in motor neurons,[38] MuSK probably acts via retrograde signals to maintain the presynaptic structures and functions. Despite the impairment of the retrograde signals caused by anti-MuSK autoantibodies, outgrowth and sprouting of axons can still be observed, suggesting a compensatory mechanism for the partial denervation in MuSK-MG patients and animal models (see **Fig. 2; Fig. 4**).[53–57]

SUMMARY

NMJs maintain a highly organized structure to achieve reliable synaptic transmission for neuromuscular functions. However, NMJs remain stable and maintain their structure for the lifetime of humans and animals. Therefore, autoimmune attack of NMJ proteins and congenital mutations of genes coding the NMJ components cause neuromuscular diseases and myasthenia syndromes.

REFERENCES

1. An X, Yue B, Lee JH, et al. Intramuscular distribution of the phrenic nerve in human diaphragm as shown by Sihler staining. Muscle Nerve 2012;45(4):522–6.
2. Sanes JR, Lichtman JW. Induction, assembly, maturation and maintenance of a postsynaptic apparatus. Nat Rev Neurosci 2001;2(11):791–805.

3. Caldwell JH. Clustering of sodium channels at the neuromuscular junction. Microsc Res Tech 2000;49(1):84–9.
4. Fambrough DM. Control of acetylcholine receptors in skeletal muscle. Physiol Rev 1979;59(1):165–227.
5. Raftery MA, Hunkapiller MW, Strader CD, et al. Acetylcholine receptor: complex of homologous subunits. Science 1980;208(4451):1454–6.
6. Unwin N. Refined structure of the nicotinic acetylcholine receptor at 4A resolution. J Mol Biol 2005;346(4):967–89.
7. Akaaboune M, Culican SM, Turney SG, et al. Rapid and reversible effects of activity on acetylcholine receptor density at the neuromuscular junction in vivo. Science 1999;286(5439):503–7.
8. Sine SM. End-plate acetylcholine receptor: structure, mechanism, pharmacology, and disease. Physiol Rev 2012;92(3):1189–234.
9. Patton BL. Basal lamina and the organization of neuromuscular synapses. J Neurocytol 2003;32(5):883–903.
10. Sanes JR. The basement membrane/basal lamina of skeletal muscle. J Biol Chem 2003;278(15):12601–4.
11. Timpl R, Brown JC. Supramolecular assembly of basement membranes. Bioessays 1996;18(2):123–32.
12. Rogers RS, Nishimune H. The role of laminins in the organization and function of neuromuscular junctions. Matrix Biol 2017;57-58:86–105.
13. Fox MA. Novel roles for collagens in wiring the vertebrate nervous system. Curr Opin Cell Biol 2008;20(5):508–13.
14. Sanes JR, Lichtman JW. Development of the vertebrate neuromuscular junction. Annu Rev Neurosci 1999;22:389–442.
15. Darabid H, Perez-Gonzalez AP, Robitaille R. Neuromuscular synaptogenesis: coordinating partners with multiple functions. Nat Rev Neurosci 2014;15(11):703–18.
16. Couteaux R, Pecot-Dechavassine M. Synaptic vesicles and pouches at the level of "active zones" of the neuromuscular junction. C R Acad Sci Hebd Seances Acad Sci D 1970;271(25):2346–9.
17. Tsuji S. Rene Couteaux (1909-1999) and the morphological identification of synapses. Biol Cell 2006;98(8):503–9.
18. Sudhof TC. The presynaptic active zone. Neuron 2012;75(1):11–25.
19. Nishimune H. Active zones of mammalian neuromuscular junctions: formation, density, and aging. Ann N Y Acad Sci 2012;1274(1):24–32.
20. Fukuoka T, Engel AG, Lang B, et al. Lambert-Eaton myasthenic syndrome: I. Early morphological effects of IgG on the presynaptic membrane active zones. Ann Neurol 1987;22(2):193–9.
21. Nishimune H, Sanes JR, Carlson SS. A synaptic laminin-calcium channel interaction organizes active zones in motor nerve terminals. Nature 2004;432(7017):580–7.
22. Kang H, Tian L, Thompson W. Terminal Schwann cells guide the reinnervation of muscle after nerve injury. J Neurocytol 2003;32(5–8):975–85.
23. Sugiura Y, Lin W. Neuron-glia interactions: the roles of Schwann cells in neuromuscular synapse formation and function. Biosci Rep 2011;31(5):295–302.
24. Ko CP, Robitaille R. Perisynaptic Schwann cells at the neuromuscular synapse: adaptable, multitasking glial cells. Cold Spring Harb Perspect Biol 2015;7(10):a020503.
25. Barik A, Li L, Sathyamurthy A, et al. Schwann cells in neuromuscular junction formation and maintenance. J Neurosci 2016;36(38):9770–81.

26. Reddy LV, Koirala S, Sugiura Y, et al. Glial cells maintain synaptic structure and function and promote development of the neuromuscular junction in vivo. Neuron 2003;40(3):563–80.
27. Kang H, Tian L, Mikesh M, et al. Terminal Schwann cells participate in neuromuscular synapse remodeling during reinnervation following nerve injury. J Neurosci 2014;34(18):6323–33.
28. Court FA, Gillingwater TH, Melrose S, et al. Identity, developmental restriction and reactivity of extralaminar cells capping mammalian neuromuscular junctions. J Cell Sci 2008;121(Pt 23):3901–11.
29. DeChiara TM, Bowen DC, Valenzuela DM, et al. The receptor tyrosine kinase MuSK is required for neuromuscular junction formation in vivo. Cell 1996;85(4): 501–12.
30. Burgess RW, Nguyen QT, Son YJ, et al. Alternatively spliced isoforms of nerve- and muscle-derived agrin: their roles at the neuromuscular junction. Neuron 1999;23(1):33–44.
31. Weatherbee SD, Anderson KV, Niswander LA. LDL-receptor-related protein 4 is crucial for formation of the neuromuscular junction. Development 2006;133(24): 4993–5000.
32. Wu H, Lu Y, Shen C, et al. Distinct roles of muscle and motoneuron LRP4 in neuromuscular junction formation. Neuron 2012;75(1):94–107.
33. Yumoto N, Kim N, Burden SJ. Lrp4 is a retrograde signal for presynaptic differentiation at neuromuscular synapses. Nature 2012;489(7416):438–42.
34. Apel ED, Roberds SL, Campbell KP, et al. Rapsyn may function as a link between the acetylcholine receptor and the agrin-binding dystrophin-associated glycoprotein complex. Neuron 1995;15(1):115–26.
35. Apel ED, Glass DJ, Moscoso LM, et al. Rapsyn is required for MuSK signaling and recruits synaptic components to a MuSK-containing scaffold. Neuron 1997;18(4):623–35.
36. Inoue A, Setoguchi K, Matsubara Y, et al. Dok-7 activates the muscle receptor kinase MuSK and shapes synapse formation. Sci Signal 2009;2(59):ra7.
37. Okada K, Inoue A, Okada M, et al. The muscle protein Dok-7 is essential for neuromuscular synaptogenesis. Science 2006;312(5781):1802–5.
38. Valenzuela DM, Stitt TN, DiStefano PS, et al. Receptor tyrosine kinase specific for the skeletal muscle lineage: expression in embryonic muscle, at the neuromuscular junction, and after injury. Neuron 1995;15(3):573–84.
39. Glass DJ, DeChiara TM, Stitt TN, et al. The receptor tyrosine kinase MuSK is required for neuromuscular junction formation and is a functional receptor for agrin. Cold Spring Harb Symp Quant Biol 1996;61:435–44.
40. Kim N, Stiegler AL, Cameron TO, et al. Lrp4 is a receptor for agrin and forms a complex with MuSK. Cell 2008;135(2):334–42.
41. Zhang B, Luo S, Wang Q, et al. LRP4 serves as a coreceptor of agrin. Neuron 2008;60(2):285–97.
42. Yamanashi Y, Tezuka T, Yokoyama K. Activation of receptor protein-tyrosine kinases from the cytoplasmic compartment. J Biochem 2012;151(4):353–9.
43. Evoli A, Tonali PA, Padua L, et al. Clinical correlates with anti-MuSK antibodies in generalized seronegative myasthenia gravis. Brain 2003;126(Pt 10):2304–11.
44. Sanders DB, El-Salem K, Massey JM, et al. Clinical aspects of MuSK antibody positive seronegative MG. Neurology 2003;60(12):1978–80.
45. Bartoccioni E, Scuderi F, Minicuci GM, et al. Anti-MuSK antibodies: correlation with myasthenia gravis severity. Neurology 2006;67(3):505–7.

46. Deymeer F, Gungor-Tuncer O, Yilmaz V, et al. Clinical comparison of anti-MuSK-vs anti-AChR-positive and seronegative myasthenia gravis. Neurology 2007; 68(8):609–11.
47. Ohta K, Shigemoto K, Fujinami A, et al. Clinical and experimental features of MuSK antibody positive MG in Japan. Eur J Neurol 2007;14(9):1029–34.
48. Evoli A, Bianchi MR, Riso R, et al. Response to therapy in myasthenia gravis with anti-MuSK antibodies. Ann N Y Acad Sci 2008;1132:76–83.
49. Wolfe GI, Oh SJ. Clinical phenotype of muscle-specific tyrosine kinase-antibody-positive myasthenia gravis. Ann N Y Acad Sci 2008;1132:71–5.
50. Oh SJ. Muscle-specific receptor tyrosine kinase antibody positive myasthenia gravis current status. J Clin Neurol 2009;5(2):53–64.
51. Pasnoor M, Wolfe GI, Nations S, et al. Clinical findings in MuSK-antibody positive myasthenia gravis: a U.S. experience. Muscle Nerve 2010;41(3):370–4.
52. Gilhus NE, Verschuuren JJ. Myasthenia gravis: subgroup classification and therapeutic strategies. Lancet Neurol 2015;14(10):1023–36.
53. Shigemoto K, Kubo S, Maruyama N, et al. Induction of myasthenia by immunization against muscle-specific kinase. J Clin Invest 2006;116(4):1016–24.
54. Cole RN, Reddel SW, Gervasio OL, et al. Anti-MuSK patient antibodies disrupt the mouse neuromuscular junction. Ann Neurol 2008;63(6):782–9.
55. Mori S, Kubo S, Akiyoshi T, et al. Antibodies against muscle-specific kinase impair both presynaptic and postsynaptic functions in a murine model of myasthenia gravis. Am J Pathol 2012;180(2):798–810.
56. Niks EH, Kuks JB, Wokke JH, et al. Pre- and postsynaptic neuromuscular junction abnormalities in musk myasthenia. Muscle Nerve 2010;42(2):283–8.
57. Viegas S, Jacobson L, Waters P, et al. Passive and active immunization models of MuSK-Ab positive myasthenia: electrophysiological evidence for pre and postsynaptic defects. Exp Neurol 2012;234(2):506–12.
58. Mori S, Kishi M, Kubo S, et al. 3,4-Diaminopyridine improves neuromuscular transmission in a MuSK antibody-induced mouse model of myasthenia gravis. J Neuroimmunol 2012;245(1–2):75–8.
59. Morsch M, Reddel SW, Ghazanfari N, et al. Pyridostigmine but not 3,4-diaminopyridine exacerbates ACh receptor loss and myasthenia induced in mice by muscle-specific kinase autoantibody. J Physiol 2013;591(Pt 10):2747–62.
60. Evoli A, Alboini PE, Damato V, et al. 3,4-Diaminopyridine may improve myasthenia gravis with MuSK antibodies. Neurology 2016;86(11):1070–1.

Ocular Myasthenia

Mohammed Al-Haidar, MD[a,b], Michael Benatar, MD, PhD[a,b],
Henry J. Kaminski, MD[a,b],*

KEYWORDS

- Myasthenia gravis • Ocular myasthenia • Ptosis • Double vision • Prednisone
- Acetylcholine receptor • Extraocular muscle

KEY POINTS

- Ocular myasthenia may be profoundly visually disabling, and its potential compromise to quality of life should not be underestimated.
- The diagnosis of ocular myasthenia needs to be considered in any patient with painless pupillary-sparing ophthalmoparesis.
- Most patients will have negative autoantibody and repetitive nerve stimulation tests.
- Most patients respond well to corticosteroids, but nonsteroid immunosuppressive agents may be necessary for those who have adverse effects or are treatment resistant.

INTRODUCTION

Myasthenia gravis (MG) has a propensity to involve the extraocular muscles (EOMs) and the levator palpebrae. Approximately half of patients will have symptoms of ocular muscle weakness as the first manifestation of MG before development of generalized weakness, whereas 15% to 49% of patients will remain with weakness restricted to the eye muscles, which defines ocular myasthenia (OM).[1,2] Importantly, because OM is defined by current symptoms and signs, a patient who previously had generalized MG, but now has solely ocular manifestations of disease, is appropriately designated as having OM. The age and sex distribution of patients with OM reflects the demography of generalized MG with a predominance of women with an onset before 40 years of age and men developing OM at older ages.[3] OM seems to be more common in Asian populations with a predilection for a juvenile onset, which is quite different from observations of European and American populations.[4–7] This review provides an overview of OM diagnosis and treatment and includes a discussion of pathogenic mechanisms that may underlie the susceptibility of ocular muscles to

[a] Department of Neurology, George Washington University, 2150 Pennsylvania Avenue, Northwest, Washington, DC 20037, USA; [b] Department of Neurology, 1150 Northwest 14th Street #715, Miami, FL 33136, USA
* Corresponding author. Department of Neurology, George Washington University, 2150 Pennsylvania Avenue, Northwest, Washington, DC 20037.
E-mail address: hkaminski@mfa.gwu.edu

Neurol Clin 36 (2018) 241–251
https://doi.org/10.1016/j.ncl.2018.01.003
0733-8619/18/© 2018 Elsevier Inc. All rights reserved.

neurologic.theclinics.com

MG. Firm recommendations regarding treatment are difficult to make given the limitations of available evidence.

REASONS FOR PREFERENTIAL OCULAR MUSCLE INVOLVEMENT IN MYASTHENIA GRAVIS

The final effector mechanism of autoantibody injury to the neuromuscular junction is likely to be shared between OM and generalized MG. Indeed, single-fiber examination of the extremity muscle of patients with OM may demonstrate impaired neuromuscular transmission supporting the hypothesis that OM is simply a less severe form of generalized disease,[8] raising the possibility that the high frequency of ocular symptoms simply reflects the sensitivity of ocular muscle function to perturbation with resulting symptoms. In an effort to understand the heightened sensitivity of ocular muscles to the disease process in MG, some have noted that the EOMs, unlike other skeletal muscles, express both the embryonic and adult isoforms of the acetylcholine receptor (AChR), suggesting perhaps that antigenic targets expressed *only* at the ocular muscle neuromuscular junctions could account for isolated injury of ocular muscle by an autoimmune attack. But targeting of the fetal receptor by autoantibodies does not seem to be an explanation for differential injury.[9]

A more likely explanation is that the EOMs have intrinsic properties that could place them at risk for a neuromuscular transmission disorder: (a) EOMs have less mature synaptic folding, which, in combination with a lower density of AChRs, would reduce the end plate potential and, thereby, lower the safety factor for neuromuscular transmission; (b) The extremely high motor neuron stimulation rate could also make EOM synapses more susceptible to failure of neuromuscular transmission[10,11]; (c) Upwards of 20% of EOM fibers have neuromuscular junctions that support tonic rather than twitch muscle contractions. Because the contractile force of these tonic fibers depend highly on the amplitude of the end plate potential, any reduction in end plate potential amplitude that results from the loss of AChR produced by MG would lead to a weaker contraction; (d) Intrinsic complement regulators protect the postsynaptic surface of the neuromuscular junction from complement-mediated damage of MG. These regulators are expressed at lower levels at EOM junctions compared with neuromuscular junctions of other muscles,[12,13] putting these junctions at greater risk for complement-mediated injury of MG.

Reasons for the susceptibility of the levator are much less well understood. When the lids are open, the levator is under repetitive activation, which may make them susceptible to transmission fatigue. Although the levator contains muscle fiber types that support fatigue resistance similar to those of EOMs, the junctional anatomy is not known to have characteristics that would suggest a susceptibility to neuromuscular transmission compromise.[14]

CLINICAL FEATURES
Symptoms

Patients typically present with any combination of painless fluctuating unilateral, bilateral, or alternating eyelid droop in combination with double vision. A history of alternating ptosis is pathognomonic for MG.[15] Symptoms usually become more pronounced toward the evening and improve with sleep or rest. Once ptosis covers the pupil, patients may appreciate blurred vision. Because of hyper-retraction of one lid, patients may complain of ocular irritation. Although double vision is the most common symptom, some patients may report dizziness or gait instability related to dysconjugate eye movements. Such symptoms should improve with covering one eye.[16] Some patients have light sensitivity, arriving at the office wearing dark glasses.

Signs

Enhancement of ptosis with sustained up-gaze is the classic examination finding of MG, and repeated lid closure and opening may also enhance ptosis. Ptosis may be unilateral or bilateral and is often asymmetric.[16] The asymmetry of ptosis may be so marked that one lid is hyper-retracted. Enhanced ptosis may be observed when the more ptotic lid is passively elevated leading to increased droop of the contralateral lid.[17] Enhanced ptosis and lid retraction relate to the Hering law of innervation, which states that each levator receives equal neuronal stimulation leading to one lid muscle receiving excess stimulation for its position.[18] The Cogan lid twitch sign is elicited by directing patients to look down for 10 seconds followed by rapid repositioning to primary gaze. The ptotic lid has a momentary upward twitch.[19] The Cogan lid twitch sign is reported to have a sensitivity of up to 75% and a specificity approaching 99%.[20] False positives are rare and can be differentiated by the lack of significant fluctuation of the lid position.

Orbicularis oculi weakness may be appreciated with forced lid closure. With initial forced closure, the lids are closed tightly; but then separation is observed and may be so severe as to lead to sclera exposure, the so-called peak sign.[21] Involvement of the orbicularis oculi is not considered a sign of generalized disease, a principle enshrined in the MG Foundation of America's clinical classification system that permits such weakness in patients with OM.[22]

Ophthalmoparesis may be present with any combination of muscle involvement, ranging from individual muscle palsy to complete external ophthalmoplegia. Ocular involvement by MG may mimic numerous oculomotor disturbances including superior oblique weakness,[23] oculomotor nerve palsy,[24] isolated inferior oblique palsy,[25] internuclear ophthalmoplegia,[26-28] chronic progressive external ophthalmoplegia,[29] one-and-a-half syndrome,[30] and double depressor palsy.[31] Apart from saccadic fatigue, which may be observed when a rapid eye movement begins to slow as it approaches a target,[32,33] normal saccadic velocity within the limited range of movement of an ophthalmoparesis is an important feature that differentiates MG from other causes of ophthalmoplegia.[34] Given the heterogeneity of the ophthalmoplegia, the diagnosis of MG should be considered in anyone with acquired painless ocular motility dysfunction. Importantly, pupillary abnormalities should always lead to consideration of other diagnoses.

Differential Diagnosis

Ocular manifestations of MG may mimic central disorders of ocular motility and ptosis; however, such pathology will typically have differentiating signs on examination. In contrast, isolated ocular cranial neuropathies may be particularly difficult to distinguish from OM unless clear fatigue is observed. A history of variability in the severity of double vision may be helpful to identify OM. Graves ophthalmopathy may present with unilateral or bilateral restricted ocular motility, but ptosis is absent. If ptosis is present in patients with Graves disease, coexistent MG must be considered.[35] Patients with OM who develop new double vision or are treatment resistant should undergo evaluation for Graves ophthalmopathy with orbital imaging. Chronic progressive external ophthalmoplegia manifesting with ptosis and ophthalmoplegia should be differentiated from MG by its gradual onset, presence of nonfluctuating symmetric ptosis, and slow saccades. Third nerve lesions, Horner syndrome, senile ptosis, and levator dehiscence are readily differentiated by the absence of significant variability of symptoms, fatigability, and associated abnormalities. Lack of variability and fatigability, or the presence of pain, abnormal pupillary function, or sensory manifestations call the diagnosis of MG into question.

DIAGNOSTIC EVALUATION

The accuracy of various tests for the diagnosis of OM is summarized in[36] and in **Table 1**. These estimates of sensitivity and specificity should be treated with some caution given the methodological limitations of the studies that have investigated their diagnostic accuracy.

Nonpharmacologic Tests

The ice pack and sleep (rest) tests are easy to perform and are considered reliable adjunct tests to support the diagnosis of OM. The ice pack test is performed by placing a cooling pack over the lids for 2 to 5 minutes and then assessing for improvement in ptosis.[45,46] For the sleep test, patients are placed in a dark quiet room, with instructions to close their lids for 30 minutes, and then evaluated for improvement in ptosis or ophthalmoparesis.[47]

Edrophonium Test

Despite its long history of diagnostic use and excellent safety record, the edrophonium test has fallen out of favor because of excessive concern for severe adverse effects with potential liability issues.[48–50] Edrophonium is a short-acting acetylcholinesterase inhibitor with an onset of action within 10 to 30 seconds of intravenous administration, noted by improvement in muscle function that typically resolves within 5 minutes.[51] An initial dose of 2 mg is given; if no positive response occurs after 45 seconds, additional 2-mg doses are administered up to a maximum of 10 mg. Once a positive result is obtained, no further injection is necessary. Adverse effects may include excess salivation, sweating, nausea, and fasciculations. Rarely, serious adverse effects, such as hypotension and bradycardia, may occur. The edrophonium test is relatively contraindicated in patients with a history of bronchial asthma and cardiac dysrhythmias.[49]

Table 1
Published reports of sensitivity and specificity of diagnostic tests

	Sensitivity (%)	Specificity (%)	Patients (No.)	Reference
Ice pack test	80	100	40	Golnik et al,[37] 1999; Evoli et al,[38] 1988
Sleep test	99	91	—	Benatar,[36] 2006
Tensilon test	88	50	138	Mittal et al,[39] 2011
	97	83	86	Padua et al,[40] 2000
AChR antibodies	44	100	86	Padua et al,[40] 2000
	70.9	—	223	Peeler et al,[41] 2015
RNS	15	89	86	Padua et al,[40] 2000
	24	100	138	Mittal et al,[39] 2011
	50	—	48	Evoli et al,[42] 2003
SFEMG	90	100	138	Mittal et al,[39] 2011
	93	100	22	Milone et al,[43] 1993
	100	67	41	Rouseev et al,[44] 1992

Abbreviations: RNS, repetitive nerve stimulation; SFEMG, single-fiber electromyography.

Autoantibody Assessment

The detection of serum AChR antibodies is essentially diagnostic for MG with only rare situations of false-positive tests among patients with thymoma or family members with MG.[52,53] However, the absence of AChR antibodies does not exclude the disease, with upwards of half of patients with OM being negative.[36] Muscle-specific kinase (MuSK) antibodies may rarely be found among patients with isolated ocular presentations and pure OM.[42,54,55] Given the significantly higher cost of MuSK testing, the authors recommend a stepwise approach, only ordering MuSK antibodies after AChR antibodies are found to be negative. It is worth remembering that those who are seronegative may have low levels of a high-affinity antibody that cannot be detected by conventional assays[52,56,57] or only low-affinity antibodies that are not detected by commercial assays.

Electrodiagnostic Tests

At most, 50% of patients with OM have abnormalities on repetitive nerve stimulation (RNS) according to published studies; but even these may be overestimates for individuals with truly isolated ocular muscle weakness.[36,39,40] Therefore, a negative RNS evaluation does not exclude the disease; consideration should be given to the use of single-fiber EMG as the primary neurophysiologic evaluation for OM. Single-fiber electromyography (EMG) is the most sensitive test for the diagnosis of OM, especially when facial muscles (frontalis, orbicularis oculi) are assessed, with sensitivity estimates ranging from 90% to 100%.[39,43,44] However, in one systematic review, the sensitivity was found to be as low as 66%[36]; in general clinical practice, sensitivity is likely lower. A drawback of single-fiber EMG is the requirement for an experienced neurophysiologist, who may not be available at all institutions or private practice clinics. Further, single-fiber examination requires cooperation of patients despite the discomfort of needle placement; but only rare patients cannot tolerate the examination.

Additional Tests

Patients diagnosed with OM need to be evaluated for comorbidities. Chest imaging is required to exclude the presence of thymoma. Because of the frequency of coexistent thyroid disorder, thyroid function tests should be performed.[35] Depending on the presentation, diagnostic studies for rheumatoid arthritis, systemic lupus erythematosus, or other autoimmune disorders may be appropriate.[58,59] In patients at high risk for latent tuberculosis, it may be prudent to consider testing (eg, interferon gold) before initiation of immune-suppressive therapy.

TREATMENT

Treatment of OM may be divided into 2 general categories: (1) symptomatic therapy with local assistive devices and acetylcholinesterase inhibitors and (2) therapy targeting the autoimmune process. **Fig. 1** depicts a general treatment approach, which must be tailored to the individual characteristics of each patient.

Assistive Devices

Ptosis crutches or tape may be helpful for some patients to alleviate lid droop[60]; however, only rare patients tolerate these and there is the potential for corneal injury from exposure. Diplopia is eliminated by visual occlusive devices, which include eye patches, spectacles with one lens blocked, or opaque contact lenses.[61] Of course, patients do lose the ipsilateral visual field. For patients with stable misalignment that

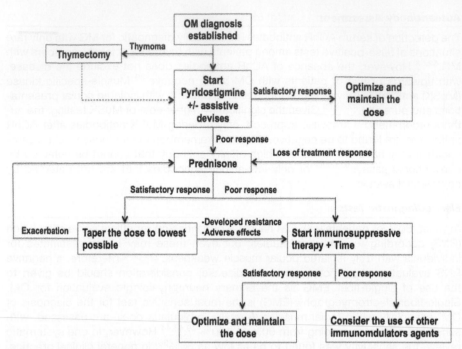

Fig. 1. General approach for treatment of OM.

is not large, prisms can be effective to limit diplopia.[62] Unfortunately, a hallmark of ocular involvement by MG is its fluctuating nature; patients presenting with a history of frequent alterations in prism prescription for double vision should be evaluated for MG.

Pharmacologic Therapy

Acetylcholinesterase inhibitors are the first line of treatment, yielding symptomatic improvement in some patients; however, they do not impact the underlying autoimmune pathology.[63] Pyridostigmine bromide is the most common preparation and is typically started at 30 to 60 mg 3 times a day with increases up to 90 to 120 mg every 3 to 4 hours based on tolerability and clinical response.[61] Ptosis responds well, but diplopia often does not given the ocular motor system's need for precise alignment. Among patients with a large separation of visual axes, symptomatic double vision may actually worsen because of an inability to ignore the false image. An apparent lack of improvement or worsening of symptoms should not necessarily lead to questioning of the diagnosis. Abdominal cramps, nausea, and diarrhea are common but can be limited with the administration of selective muscarinic antagonists, such as propantheline and glycopyrrolate; however, this complicates the patients' drug regimen. Cholinesterase inhibition proves inadequate for most patients,[64] but upwards of 30% may have relief for episodic exacerbations.[65]

Most patients with OM will require corticosteroid therapy. The use of steroids to treat OM has historically relied mostly on anecdotal data. More recently, data from a small randomized controlled trial provide evidence that low-dose prednisone, initiated at 10 mg every other day, and gradually titrated up every 2 weeks to a maximum of 40 mg per day over 16 weeks, is highly effective.[66] There were enrollment challenges in this study, as 11 out of 88 planned subjects entered the study and were randomized. However, this is the best placebo-controlled trial in OM, as it demonstrated significant benefits of prednisone despite low enrollment. The primary outcome measure was treatment failure, and all 5 placebo-treated subjects experienced that, compared with only 1 of 6 subjects in the prednisone-treated group. In this trial, median time to minimal manifestation status was 14 weeks, with patients requiring a median prednisone dose of 15 mg/d, range 15 to 25 mg per day.[66] Responders were able to taper prednisone dose to 10 to 15 mg per day without symptom relapse. Discontinuation of prednisone may lead to exacerbation, and a decision to maintain therapy at a low dose should be made with patients. Retrospective studies suggest that patients treated with corticosteroids have a higher incidence of remission, clinical improvement, and a lower risk of conversion to generalized MG.[1,51,64,67,68] However, there is a subset of patients with treatment-resistant OM or who have contraindications to corticosteroids who will require nonsteroid immunosuppressive therapy.[69]

Mycophenolate mofetil and azathioprine have been investigated as sole therapies for OM. A prospective observational study examined the efficacy of mycophenolate in 31 patients with pure OM and found that 25 of 27 patients who remained on mycophenolate did not develop generalized MG and had no significant adverse effects.[70] The standard dose of mycophenolate is 1000 mg twice daily.[62] A retrospective study of patients with OM treated with azathioprine as either a monotherapy or in combination with steroids, thymectomy, or both suggested a reduction of conversion to generalized MG, alleviation of ocular symptoms, and induction of remission.[71] The azathioprine dose is initially targeted based on weight (2.5-3.0 mg/kg/d). Tacrolimus and cyclosporine, which are used for generalized MG, may be considered in rare patients with OM when corticosteroids and other immunomodulators have failed. Plasma exchange has not been investigated for the treatment of OM, whereas a double-blind randomized placebo-controlled trial of intravenous immunoglobulin (IVIG) that evaluated 17 patients with OM found no benefit.[72] Given the paucity of evidence to support the use of IVG or plasma exchange in OM, and their potential for significant side effects, the authors do not recommend their use for OM.

Surgical Intervention

Two studies that examined the effects of thymectomy on patients with OM showed no improvement of symptoms or reduction in risk of progression to generalized MG.[73,74] The authors do not recommend thymectomy for OM, unless a thymoma is suspected.

Blepharoplasty may be considered for chronic severely disabling ptosis that is refractory to medical therapy. Reports describe satisfactory results with such a procedure[75–77]; but the authors would only recommend surgery for patients with chronic, stable lid droop. Strabismus surgery may be performed on select patients with diplopia who have had a stable angle of deviation, as assessed by an ophthalmologist, for at least 6 months.[60,78–80]

SUMMARY

OM can be a challenging condition to identify clinically and rigorously confirm its diagnosis. The authors' experience indicates that patients with chronic progressive external ophthalmoplegia or familial ptosis are the ones most often misdiagnosed with OM, whereas failure to diagnose OM is much more common. OM needs to be considered in patients with fluctuating unilateral or bilateral ptosis and among those with any pattern of painless pupil sparing ophthalmoparesis. The clinician must be aware of the numerous false-negative serologic and neurophysiologic evaluations that occur among patients with OM. The goal of therapy is to restore a normal state of vision, and the therapeutic armamentarium includes many options. Corticosteroids are highly effective, but their use must be tempered by their potential for side effects. It is currently unknown whether early immunosuppressive therapy reduces the risk of progression to generalized MG.

REFERENCES

1. Grob D, Arsura EL, Brunner NG, et al. The course of myasthenia gravis and therapies affecting outcome. Ann N Y Acad Sci 1987;505:472–99.
2. Bever CT, Aquino AV, Penn AS, et al. Prognosis of ocular myasthenia. Ann Neurol 1983;14:516–9.
3. Grob D, Brunner N, Namba T, et al. Lifetime course of myasthenia gravis. Muscle Nerve 2008;37:141–9.
4. Chiu H-C, Vincent A, Newsom-Davis J, et al. Myasthenia gravis: population differences in disease expression and acetylcholine receptor antibody titers between Chinese and Caucasians. Neurology 1987;37:1854.
5. Hawkins BR, Yu YL, Wong V, et al. Possible evidence for a variant of myasthenia gravis based on HLA and acetylcholine receptor antibody in Chinese patients. Q J Med 1989;70:235–41.
6. Wong V, Hawkins BR, Yu YL. Myasthenia gravis in Hong Kong Chinese: 2. Paediatric disease. Acta Neurol Scand 1992;86:68–72.
7. Zhang X, Yang M, Xu J, et al. Clinical and serological study of myasthenia gravis in HuBei Province, China. J Neurol Neurosurg Psychiatry 2006;78:386–90.
8. Cui L-Y, Guan Y-Z, Liu M-S, et al. Single-fiber electromyography in the extensor digitorum communis for the predictive prognosis of ocular myasthenia gravis: a retrospective study of 102 cases. Chin Med J 2015;128:2783–6.
9. Kaminski HJ, Kusner LL, Block CH. Expression of acetylcholine receptor isoforms at extraocular muscle endplates. Invest Ophthalmol Vis Sci 1996;37:345–51.
10. Kaminski HJ, Li Z, Richmonds C, et al. Susceptibility of ocular tissues to autoimmune diseases. Ann N Y Acad Sci 2003;998:362–74.
11. Kaminski HJ, Maas E, Spiegel P, et al. Why are eye muscles frequently involved in myasthenia gravis? Neurology 1990;40:1663–9.
12. Soltys J, Gong B, Kaminski HJ, et al. Extraocular muscle susceptibility to myasthenia gravis. Ann N Y Acad Sci 2008;1132:220–4.
13. Kaminski H, Li Z, Richmonds C, et al. Complement regulators in extraocular muscle and experimental autoimmune myasthenia gravis. Exp Neurol 2004;189:333–42.
14. Porter JD, Burns LA, May PJ. Morphological substrate for eyelid movements: innervation and structure of primate levator palpebrae superioris and orbicularis oculi muscles. J Comp Neurol 1989;287:64–81.
15. Osserman KE. Ocular myasthenia gravis. Invest Ophthalmol 1967;6:277–87.
16. Kusner LL, Puwanant A, Kaminski HJ. Ocular myasthenia: diagnosis, treatment, and pathogenesis. Neurologist 2006;12:231–9.
17. Gorelick PB, Rosenberg M, Pagano RJ. Enhanced ptosis in myasthenia gravis. Arch Neurol 1981;38:531.
18. Gay AJ, Salmon ML, Windsor CE. Hering's law, the levators, and their relationship in disease states. Arch Ophthalmol 1967;77:157–60.
19. Cogan DG. Myasthenia gravis: a review of the disease and a description of lid twitch as a characteristic sign. Arch Ophthalmol 1965;74:217–21.

20. Singman EL, Matta NS, Silbert DI. Use of the Cogan lid twitch to identify myasthenia gravis. J Neuroophthalmol 2011;31:239–40.
21. Osher RH. Orbicularis fatigue. Arch Ophthalmol 1979;97:677–9.
22. Jaretzki A, Barohn RJ, Ernstoff RM, et al. Myasthenia gravis: recommendations for clinical research standards. Neurology 2000;55:16–23.
23. Rush JA, Shafrin F. Ocular myasthenia presenting as superior oblique weakness. J Clin Neuroophthalmol 1982;2:125–7.
24. Appenzeller S, Veilleux M, Clarke A. Third cranial nerve palsy or pseudo 3rd nerve palsy of myasthenia gravis? A challenging diagnosis in systemic lupus erythematosus. Lupus 2009;18:836–40.
25. Almog Y, Ben-David M, Nemet AY. Inferior oblique muscle paresis as a sign of myasthenia gravis. J Clin Neurosci 2015;25:50–3.
26. Glaser JS. Myasthenic psuedointernuclear ophthalmoplegia. Arch Ophthalmol 1966;75:363–6.
27. Jay WM, Nazarian SM, Underwood DW. Pseudo-internuclear ophthalmoplegia with downshoot in myasthenia gravis. J Clin Neuroophthalmol 1987;7:74–6.
28. Argyriou AA, Karanasios P, Potsios C, et al. Myasthenia gravis initially presenting with pseudo-internuclear ophthalmoplegia. Neurol Sci 2009;30:387–8.
29. Das JC, Chaudhuri Z, Bhomaj S, et al. Ocular myasthenia presenting as progressive external ophthalmoplegia. J Pediatr Ophthalmol Strabismus 2002;39:52–4.
30. Bandini F, Faga D, Simonetti S. Ocular myasthenia mimicking a one-and-a-half syndrome. J Neuroophthalmol 2001;21:210–1.
31. Lee K, Kim US. A case of ocular myasthenia gravis presenting as double depressor palsy. Korean J Ophthalmol 2014;28:194–6.
32. Baloh RW, Keesey JC. Saccade fatigue and response to edrophonium for the diagnosis of myasthenia gravis. Ann N Y Acad Sci 1976;274:631–41.
33. Metz HS, Scott AB, O'meara DM. Saccadic eye movements in myasthenia gravis. Arch Ophthalmol 1972;88:9–11.
34. Cogan DG. Rapid eye movements in myasthenia gravis. Arch Ophthalmol 1976;94:1083–5.
35. Sahay BM, Blendis LM, Greene R. Relation between myasthenia gravis and thyroid disease. Br Med J 1965;(5437):762–5.
36. Benatar M. A systematic review of diagnostic studies in myasthenia gravis. Neuromuscul Disord 2006;16:459–67.
37. Golnik KC, Pena R, Lee AG, et al. An ice test for the diagnosis of myasthenia gravis. Ophthalmology 1999;106:1282–6.
38. Evoli A, Tonali P, Bartoccioni E, et al. Ocular myasthenia: diagnostic and therapeutic problems. Acta Neurol Scand 1988;77:31–5.
39. Mittal MK, Barohn RJ, Pasnoor M, et al. Ocular myasthenia gravis in an academic neuro-ophthalmology clinic: clinical features and therapeutic response. J Clin Neuromuscul Dis 2011;13:46–52.
40. Padua L, Stalberg E, Lomonaco M, et al. SFEMG in ocular myasthenia gravis diagnosis. Clin Neurophysiol 2000;111:1203–7.
41. Peeler CE, Lott LBD, Nagia L, et al. Clinical utility of acetylcholine receptor antibody testing in ocular myasthenia gravis. JAMA Neurol 2015;72:1170–4.
42. Evoli A, Tonali PA, Padua L, et al. Clinical correlates with anti-MuSK antibodies in generalized seronegative myasthenia gravis. Brain 2003;126:2304–11.
43. Milone M, Monaco ML, Evoli A, et al. Ocular myasthenia: diagnostic value of single fibre EMG in the orbicularis oculi muscle. J Neurol Neurosurg Psychiatry 1993;56:720–1.

44. Rouseev R, Ashby P, Basinski A, et al. Single fiber EMG in the frontalis muscle in ocular myasthenia: specificity and sensitivity. Muscle Nerve 1992;15:399–403.

45. Mahajan SK, Singh JB, Gupta P, et al. Ice pack test in myasthenia gravis. J Assoc Physicians India 2014;62:516–7.

46. Larner A. The place of the ice pack test in the diagnosis of myasthenia gravis. Int J Clin Pract 2004;58:887–8.

47. Odel JG, Winterkorn JM, Behrens MM. The sleep test for myasthenia gravis. A safe alternative to Tensilon. J Clin Neuroophthalmol 1991;11:288–92.

48. Ing EB, Ing SY, Ing T, et al. The complication rate of edrophonium testing for suspected myasthenia gravis. Can J Ophthalmol 2000;35:141–5.

49. Seybold ME. The office Tensilon test for ocular myasthenia gravis. Arch Neurol 1986;43:842–3.

50. Daroff RB. The office Tensilon test for ocular myasthenia gravis. Arch Neurol 1986;43:843–4.

51. Kupersmith MJ, Latkany R, Homel P. Development of generalized disease at 2 years in patients with ocular myasthenia gravis. Arch Neurol 2003;60:243–8.

52. Vincent A, Newsom-Davis J. Acetylcholine receptor antibody as a diagnostic test for myasthenia gravis: results in 153 validated cases and 2967 diagnostic assays. J Neurol Neurosurg Psychiatry 1985;48:1246–52.

53. Jacobson DM. Acetylcholine receptor antibodies in patients with graves' ophthalmopathy. J Neuroophthalmol 1995;15:166–70.

54. Zagar M, Vranjes D, Sostarko M, et al. Myasthenia gravis patients with anti-musk antibodies. Coll Antropol 2009;4:1151–4.

55. Bennett DLH, Mills KR, Riordan-Eva P, et al. Anti-MuSK antibodies in a case of ocular myasthenia gravis. J Neurol Neurosurg Psychiatry 2006;77:564–5.

56. Conti-Fine BM, Milani M, Kaminski HJ. Myasthenia gravis: past, present, and future. J Clin Invest 2006;116:2843–54.

57. Kamada M, Nakane S, Matsui N, et al. Ocular myasthenia gravis with anti-muscle-specific tyrosine kinase antibodies: two new cases and a systematic literature review. Clin Exp Neuroimmunol 2016;7:168–73.

58. Thorlacius S, Aarli JA, Riise T, et al. Associated disorders in myasthenia gravis: autoimmune diseases and their relation to thymectomy. Acta Neurol Scand 1989;80:290–5.

59. Christensen PB, Jensen TS, Tsiropoulos I, et al. Associated autoimmune disease in myasthenia gravis. Acta Neurol Scand 1995;91:192–5.

60. Lee J. Management of selected forms of neurogenic strabismus. In: Rosenbaum L, Santiago AP, editors. Clinical strabismus management. 1st edition. Philadelphia: W. B. Saunders; 1999. p. 380–92, 100.

61. Luchanok U, Kaminski HJ. Ocular myasthenia: diagnostic and treatment recommendations and the evidence base. Curr Opin Neurol 2008;21:8–15.

62. Haines SR, Thurtell MJ. Treatment of ocular myasthenia gravis. Curr Treat Options Neurol 2012;14:103–12.

63. Kupersmith MJ. Ocular myasthenia gravis: treatment successes and failures in patients with long-term follow-up. J Neurol 2009;256:1314–20.

64. Kupersmith MJ. Ocular motor dysfunction and ptosis in ocular myasthenia gravis: effects of treatment. Br J Ophthalmol 2005;89:1330–4.

65. Bhanushali MJ, Wuu J, Benatar M. Treatment of ocular symptoms in myasthenia gravis. Neurology 2008;71:1335–41.

66. Benatar M, Mcdermott MP, Sanders DB, et al. Efficacy of prednisone for the treatment of ocular myasthenia (EPITOME): a randomized, controlled trial. Muscle Nerve 2016;53:363–9.

67. Kupersmith MJ, Moster M, Bhuiyan S, et al. Beneficial effects of corticosteroids on ocular myasthenia gravis. Arch Neurol 1996;53:802–4.
68. Monsul NT, Patwa HS, Knorr AM, et al. The effect of prednisone on the progression from ocular to generalized myasthenia gravis. J Neurol Sci 2004;217:131–3.
69. Kaminski HJ, Daroff RB. Treatment of ocular myasthenia: steroids only when compelled. Arch Neurol 2000;57:752–3.
70. Chan JW. Mycophenolate mofetil for ocular myasthenia. J Neurol 2008;255: 510–3.
71. Sommer N, Sigg B, Melms A, et al. Ocular myasthenia gravis: response to long-term immunosuppressive treatment. J Neurol Neurosurg Psychiatry 1997;62: 156–62.
72. Zinman L, Ng E, Bril V. IV immunoglobulin in patients with myasthenia gravis: a randomized controlled trial. Neurology 2007;68:837–41.
73. Kawaguchi N, Kuwabara S, Nemoto Y, et al. Treatment and outcome of myasthenia gravis: retrospective multi-center analysis of 470 Japanese patients, 1999–2000. J Neurol Sci 2004;224:43–7.
74. Papatestas AE, Genkins G, Kornfeld P, et al. Effects of thymectomy in myasthenia gravis. Ann Surg 1987;206:79–88.
75. Shimizu Y, Suzuki S, Nagasao T, et al. Surgical treatment for medically refractory myasthenic blepharoptosis. Clin Ophthalmol 2014;8:1859–67.
76. Litwin AS, Patel B, Mcnab AA, et al. Blepharoptosis surgery in patients with myasthenia gravis. Br J Ophthalmol 2015;99:899–902.
77. Lai CS, Lai YW, Huang SH, et al. Surgical correction of the intractable blepharoptosis in patients with ocular myasthenia gravis. Ann Plast Surg 2016;76(Suppl 1): S55–9.
78. Morris OC, Oday J. Strabismus surgery in the management of diplopia caused by myasthenia gravis. Br J Ophthalmol 2004;88:832.
79. Peragallo JH, Velez FG, Demer JL, et al. Long-term follow-up of strabismus surgery for patients with ocular myasthenia gravis. J Neuroophthalmol 2013;33: 40–4.
80. Acheson JF, Elston JS, Lee JP, et al. Extraocular muscle surgery in myasthenia gravis. Br J Ophthalmol 1991;75:232–5.

Generalized Myasthenia Gravis

Classification, Clinical Presentation, Natural History, and Epidemiology

Michael K. Hehir, MD[a],*, Nicholas J. Silvestri, MD[b]

KEYWORDS

- Myasthenia gravis • Acetylcholine receptor • Antimuscle-specific kinase • Occular

KEY POINTS

- Myasthenia gravis (MG) is a rare disease.
- A common yet nonspecific feature of MG is the fluctuating nature of weakness that patients experience, a phenomenon referred to as fatigability.
- The majority of patients with MG first present with ocular symptoms.
- Most patients with MG will experience at least 1 exacerbation of symptoms throughout the course of their illness.

Myasthenia gravis (MG) is the most common disorder of the neuromuscular junction. It is the prototypic autoimmune disease most commonly caused by antibodies to the acetylcholine receptor (AChR) leading to characteristic fatigable weakness of the ocular, bulbar, respiratory, axial, and limb muscles. This article will cover the epidemiology, clinical presentation, classification, and natural history of MG.

EPIDEMIOLOGY

MG is a rare disease. Wide variability in reported incidence rates (IRs) and prevalence rates (PRs) are based on several epidemiologic studies performed primarily in Europe and the United States over the past 70 years.[1–3] In general, both IR and PR are increasing in nonlinear fashion over time. The biggest increase occurred around 1980. These increases are attributed to greater awareness of the disease and improvements in diagnostic antibody testing, epidemiologic methodology, and treatment of the disease leading to better survival. Meta-analyses estimate the IR between

a Department of Neurosciences, Larner College of Medicine at the University of Vermont, University of Vermont, 1 South Prospect Street, Burlington, VT 05401, USA; b Department of Neurology, University at Buffalo Jacobs School of Medicine & Biomedical Sciences, 1010 Main Street, Buffalo, New York 14202, USA
* Corresponding author.
E-mail address: Michael.hehir@uvmhealth.org

Neurol Clin 36 (2018) 253–260
https://doi.org/10.1016/j.ncl.2018.01.002
0733-8619/18/© 2018 Elsevier Inc. All rights reserved.

5 to 30 cases per million person years.[2,3] Prevalence is estimated between 10 to 20 cases per 100,000 population; this rate is predicted to increase over time due to improved treatment and survival.[1]

There is a bimodal age distribution in the incidence of MG, with a peak around the age of 30 years and again at the age of 50 years, with a steady rise in incidence thereafter.[4,5] There is a higher frequency of females in the younger age group, which is typical of autoimmune disorders and a slightly higher frequency seen in men in the older age group.[6] Juvenile MG is defined as disease with onset before the age of 18 years and accounts for roughly 10% of all cases of MG.[1] It is more commonly reported in East Asia with a high frequency of ocular disease.[7] There is otherwise a relatively equal geographic distribution in the incidence and prevalence of MG in both adults and children. Although all ethnicities are affected by MG, there is a slightly higher prevalence among people of African descent, especially in antimuscle-specific kinase (MuSK) antibody-positive disease.[8,9] MuSK antibody-positive disease also appears to be more common in geographic locations closer to the equator.[10]

CLINICAL PRESENTATION

A common yet nonspecific feature of MG is the fluctuating nature of weakness that patients experience, a phenomenon referred to as fatigability. Patients will typically report worsening of symptoms with exercise or as the day goes on, indicative of a reduced safety factor in neuromuscular transmission due to the loss of functioning AChRs.

Patients with MG also have a distinctive pattern of weakness due to the selective vulnerability of certain muscle groups in this disorder. Most patients-roughly two-thirds-initially present with ocular symptoms: ptosis and/or diplopia without pupillary abnormalities.[11] Weakness of the eye muscles is often asymmetrical and variable. Whereas lesions of cranial nerves III, IV, or VI lead to reliable patterns of diplopia, patients with MG will often experience a combination of horizontal, vertical, or diagonal diplopia. Similarly, the degree of ptosis and eye involved can change dramatically over time. Multiple bedside maneuvers can be performed to confirm fatigable ocular weakness including sustained horizontal and vertical gaze, evaluation for Cogan lid twitch, and evaluation for a curtain sign.[12]

About 75% of patients will develop generalized weakness, typically within the first 2 to 3 years following presentation; generalization may be more rapid in anti-MuSK MG.[6,13,14] When disease becomes generalized, there is a predilection for bulbar, neck, and proximal limb muscle involvement.[11,15,16] Approximately 10% to 15% of patients can present with bulbar dysfunction.[11] Patients may develop difficulty chewing due to jaw fatigue as a meal progresses. Similarly, swallowing may be affected because of weakness of pharyngeal or tongue muscles, with dysphagia for liquids occurring more commonly than for solids. Because of a predilection for soft palate involvement, some patients describe nasal regurgitation of fluid or coughing fits after eating or drinking, the latter due to aspiration. Dysarthria is manifest by fatigable nasal, lingual, guttural, and/or labial dysarthria, or dysphonia, in contrast to the spastic dysarthria of amyotrophic lateral sclerosis. Fatigability of speech can be assessed in the clinic by asking a patient to count out loud to 50 or 100. Bifacial weakness can result in expressionless facial expression, trouble smiling, trouble whistling, and inability to fully close the eyelids.[12] Lack of facial expression can be a source of social distress for patients. Neck flexion weakness predominates in MG.[12] Rare patients can present with head drop due to neck extensor weakness; this presentation is more common in anti-MuSK MG.[13,15] When limb weakness occurs, there is preferential involvement of proximal muscles, which may affect a patient's ability to raise his or her arms, climb stairs, or rise from low chairs.

Respiratory muscle weakness can occur in up to 40% of MG patients leading to dyspnea with exertion or orthopnea.[11] Roughly 15% to 20% of patients with MG will experience myasthenic crisis, defined as respiratory failure necessitating either noninvasive positive pressure ventilation or mechanical ventilation until clinical improvement occurs; myasthenic crisis is more common in anti-MuSK MG.[11,13,17] Respiratory muscle weakness is typically associated with concurrent bulbar and neck muscle weakness.[18] In the specialized neuromuscular clinic, pulmonology clinic, or inpatient hospital unit, pulmonary function tests including forced vital capacity (FVC), mean inspiratory pressure (MIP), and mean expiratory pressure (MEP) can be measured.[19] An FVC less than 20 mL/kg and an MIP or MEP less than 40 cm/H_2O are associated with impending myasthenic crisis.[19] At the bedside, measurement of neck flexion strength and maximal counting in a single breath also have good predictive value of impending crisis.[18]

CLASSIFICATION

Due to implications for management, myasthenia gravis is classified by clinical status (ocular vs generalized disease), disease severity, antibody type, and any associated thymic pathology.[15] Pure ocular MG resulting in ptosis and/or diplopia occurs in approximately 20% of cases, and generalized MG occurs in the remainder.[6,11] Although patients with generalized MG will require treatment with immunosuppressants, many ocular MG patients can be managed with acetylcholinesterase inhibitors alone.[12,15,20] Because of the debilitating nature of ocular muscle dysfunction, immunosuppression may be needed in patients with ocular MG who fail acetylcholinesterase monotherapy.[21] In a study of 11 subjects, incidence of treatment failure was lower in the prednisone group than in the placebo group (17% vs 100%), with median time to sustained minimal manifestation status of 14 weeks while requiring an average prednisone dose of 15 mg per day.

All patients diagnosed with MG should undergo imaging (either computed tomography or MRI) of the chest to evaluate for thymic disease. Thymoma is discovered following the diagnosis of MG in 10% to 15% of patients; most have AChR antibodies and generalized disease.[6] Conversely, 30% of patients with a known thymoma develop MG.[22] Thymic lymphoid follicular hyperplasia occurs in approximately 70% of patients with generalized MG and is associated with negative imaging studies.[22,23] MG associated with higher-stage thymoma tends to have a more severe course; thymectomy is indicated in these patients.[15] Thymic hyperplasia is more common in younger patients.[16] A recent randomized control trial demonstrated clinical improvement with thymectomy in AChR antibody-positive patients without thymoma.[24]

Antibody type associated with MG also has implications for treatment and prognosis.[16] Most often MG antibodies directed against AChR (either binding, blocking, or modulating antibodies) are observed in 85% of cases of generalized MG and between 30% to 50% cases of ocular MG.[6,16] Acetylcholine binding receptor antibodies are highly specific for MG. AChR antibody titers do not generally correlate with disease severity, but titer decline is often observed when MG improves.[25]

Antibodies to MuSK occur in approximately 7% cases of generalized disease and almost never in ocular disease.[13] Anti-MuSK antibody MG is associated with early involvement of bulbar muscles, neck extensor muscles, and respiratory muscles.[13,14] Anti-MuSK MG also tends to have a more severe phenotype when compared with anti-AChR MG; about 30% of anti-MuSK MG patients will experience MG crisis.[13,14]

Thymic pathology is uncommon in anti-MuSK MG; thymectomy does not appear to be associated with improved clinical outcomes in anti-MuSK MG.[14,23,26,27] It is difficult to ascertain if thymectomy is the cause of patients' improvement, as MuSK MG cases are treated sequentially with multiple immunosuppressive agents.[13] Unlike AChR antibody MG, anti-MuSK MG patients do not typically improve with acetylcholinesterase inhibitor treatment; in some instances acetylcholinesterase inhibition may worsen weakness in anti-MuSK MG.[27] Intravenous immunoglobulin is also a less effective treatment in anti-MuSK MG.[13,27,28] Many patients with anti-MuSK MG require high doses of corticosteroids in combination with another treatment (eg, plasma exchange) to improve and maintain muscle strength.[13,14] Rituximab is emerging as a successful treatment strategy in anti-MuSK MG.[27,29]

More recently, antibodies to low-density lipoprotein receptor-related protein 4 (LRP4), agrin, and cortactin have been discovered in patients with MG.[30-33] When none of the aforementioned antibodies are detected, patients are diagnosed with MG by clinical or electrodiagnostic means (typically with single-fiber electromyography) and are termed seronegative.[34] About 7% of generalized MG patients are seronegative compared with between 50% and 70% of ocular MG patients.[12,16] Seronegative patients usually have an identical phenotype to AChR antibody MG patients.[15] Cell-based assays used to detect clustered AChR antibodies have been found to be useful in making a diagnosis of MG when conventional testing with radioimmunoprecipitation assay has been negative.[35] Patients with isolated clustered AChR antibodies tend to be younger and have higher percentage of ocular MG, milder disease without respiratory failure, and better response to treatment.[36] Further discovery of pathogenic antibodies and improvements in antibody detection are likely to decrease the percentage of patients found to have seronegative MG in the future.

Anti-LRP-4 antibodies have been discovered in 2% to 27% of MG patients without antibodies to AChR or MuSK; cases of concurrent AChR/LRP4 and MuSK/LRP4 are also described.[33] Pure LRP4 MG is associated with a more mild phenotype of MG, similar response to treatment as anti-AChR MG patients, and young female predominance.[33] The clinical presentation of double seropositive (AChR/LRP4 or MuSK/LRP4) resembles the clinical presentation of AChR or MuSK MG respectively.[33]

Antiagrin antibodies have also been demonstrated in patients with generalized MG and concurrent antibodies to AChR or MuSK.[30] The patients had a phenotype of typical ocular and generalized MG. Anticortactin antibodies have been measured in a subset of primarily seronegative female MG patients younger than age 50 with a clinical phenotype similar to AChR MG.[32] The clinical utility of these antibodies is currently under investigation.

Although they are not in and of themselves diagnostic for MG, titin and ryanodine receptor antibodies have been discovered in some patients with AChR-positive MG. The pathogenicity of these antibodies has been debated, and they are likely merely disease markers with a high prevalence in patients with concurrent thymoma.[37,38]

Juvenile MG deserves special attention as it is a unique subset of the disease. Approximately 11% to 24% of all MG patients have disease onset in childhood or adolescence.[39] Disease onset is usually after 10 years of age, and disease manifestations appear before puberty in half of cases. Onset before 1 year of age is rare.[40] Pubertal status might affect the clinical presentation, with a higher incidence of ocular MG in prepubertal patients and generalized MG in postpubertal patients.[41] Female predominance was observed only after the age of 10 years.[42] As in adult-onset cases, the disease may be generalized at onset, but isolated ocular involvement is a more common presentation followed by generalization within the next 1 to 2 years. However, children with ocular MG are more likely than adults to remain with purely ocular disease. In adults, it was thought that 85% of adults with ocular MG develop generalized disease, although more recent data from a neuro-ophthalmology clinic standpoint suggest progression from ocular MG to generalized MG occurs in only 12% of cases during mean follow-up of 3 years. [43] In children, this percentage is also ranges anywhere from 23% to 75%.[40,44,45] The occurrence of thymoma is rare.[40] The spontaneous remission rate in juvenile cases is higher than in adults and has been reported to range from 15% to 35%.[28,41,46]

Transient neonatal MG occurs in 10% to 15% of children born to mothers with the disease and is caused by transfer of antibodies across the placenta.[11] The weakness can lead to weak cry, weak suck, poor feeding, or respiratory difficulties, as well as generalized hypotonia and rarely arthrogryposis. The symptoms typically last days to a few weeks and are treatable with acetylcholinesterase inhibitors. There is no correlation with the incidence of transient neonatal MG and mother's disease severity or AChR antibody titer, and it is thought to occur because of differences in AChR epitopes, binding affinity, or other factors.[47]

MG patients can also be classified by response to treatment. Although many patients are able to live productive lives with few or no symptoms when adequately treated, there is a distinct subset of patients with aggressive and difficult-to-control disease.[48] The 2016 international consensus guidelines define refractory MG as patients with MG who have an MGFA postintervention status that is unchanged or worse after treatment with corticosteroids and at least 2 other immunosuppressant agents, used in adequate doses for an adequate duration, with persistence of symptoms or side effects that limit functioning, as defined by patient and physician.[49] The exact prevalence of refractory myasthenia is unknown, but it is estimated to occur in approximately 10% of patients with AChR-generalized MG.[50] More aggressive immune-based treatment is warranted to prevent life-threatening crises in patients with refractory MG. Although there are no evidence-based guidelines, agents such as rituximab, high dose cyclophosphamide, and more recently eculizimab may be reasonable treatments for these patients.[48,51] Thymectomy, in some cases repeat thymectomy, may also be considered in these patients.[48]

NATURAL HISTORY

As discussed previously, most patients with MG first present with ocular symptoms. Of these, 12% to 80% will develop generalized disease, with roughly 90% of cases doing so within the 2 to 3 years after diagnosis.[6,43] In the majority of patients, no precipitating factors prior to disease onset can be identified, but infections, stress, trauma, metabolic derangements, medications (eg, penicillamine), and pregnancy have all been implicated in a minority. With improved treatments, disease severity tends to lessen after the first 5 years of illness.[6]

Most patients with MG will experience at least 1 exacerbation of symptoms throughout the course of their illness. These exacerbations may be triggered by an infection (commonly an upper respiratory tract infection), a reduction in dose of medications used to treat myasthenia, the use of high-dose steroids (within the first 10–14 days) in severe or bulbar MG, administration of medications known to aggravate myasthenia, warmer ambient temperatures, or emotional stress.

As discussed previously, MG crisis occurs in approximately 15% to 20% of patients with MG and is more likely to early on in disease course, usually within the first 3 years following diagnosis.[17] Approximately 30% of patients with anti-MuSK MG experience an MG crisis; almost 70% of these crises occur within 6 months of symptom onset.[27] Myasthenic crisis treatment is aimed at identifying and treating any underlying precipitants, protection of the airway and mechanical ventilation until strength improves, and often plasmapheresis or possibly intravenous immunoglobulin.[49,52,53] The average duration of intubation is 5 days.[54] The mortality rate in myasthenic crisis is less than 5% and is usually caused by complications of hospitalization and treatment.[54]

Remission in MG can occur either with or without the need for continued treatment.[55] In his early studies examining the course of MG, Grob found that approximately 20% of patients experience a complete or nearly complete remission lasting at least 6 months.[56,57] Follow-up studies suggest a long-term remission rate of about 10%.[6] Any residual weakness tends to be confined to the orbicularis oculi. He found that although most patients have 1 remission, as many as 5% may have 2 to 4 remissions throughout the course of their disease. Most remissions occur in the first year following diagnosis but can occur much later, and the average interval between disease onset and remission is 4 years. Remission is more common in juvenile and female patients.[6]

Although the mortality rate was previously high, resulting in the name myasthenia gravis, the current mortality rate in MG is reported as 0.06 to 0.89 deaths per million person years.[3] Mortality statistics for MG have fallen dramatically over time. Between 1940 and 1957, the mortality rate was 31%, whereas between 1966 and 1985, the mortality rate was 7%.[6] The 2 primary reasons for this reduced mortality rate are the improvement in intensive respiratory care and the introduction of immunosuppressive treatments.

REFERENCES

1. Phillips LH 2nd. The epidemiology of myasthenia gravis. Ann New York Acad Sci 2003;998:407–12.
2. McGrogan A, Sneddon S, de Vries CS. The incidence of myasthenia gravis: a systematic literature review. Neuroepidemiology 2010;34:171–83.
3. Carr AS, Cardwell CR, McCarron PO, et al. A systematic review of population based epidemiological studies in myasthenia gravis. BMC Neurol 2010;10:46.
4. Heldal AT, Owe JF, Gilhus NE, et al. Seropositive myasthenia gravis: a nationwide epidemiologic study. Neurology 2009;73:150–1.
5. Andersen JB, Engeland A, Owe JF, et al. Myasthenia gravis requiring pyridostigmine treatment in a national population cohort. Eur J Neurol 2010;17:1445–50.
6. Grob D, Brunner N, Namba T, et al. Lifetime course of myasthenia gravis. Muscle Nerve 2008;37:141–9.
7. Yu YL, Hawkins BR, Ip MS, et al. Myasthenia gravis in Hong Kong Chinese. 1. epidemiology and adult disease. Acta Neurol Scand 1992;86:113–9.
8. Phillips LH 2nd, Torner JC, Anderson MS, et al. The epidemiology of myasthenia gravis in central and western Virginia. Neurology 1992;42:1888–93.
9. Oh SJ, Morgan MB, Lu L, et al. Racial differences in myasthenia gravis in Alabama. Muscle Nerve 2009;39:328–32.
10. Deymeer F, Gungor-Tuncer O, Yilmaz V, et al. Clinical comparison of anti-MuSK-vs anti-AChR-positive and seronegative myasthenia gravis. Neurology 2007;68:609–11.
11. Grob D, Arsura EL, Brunner NG, et al. The course of myasthenia gravis and therapies affecting outcome. Ann New York Acad Sci 1987;505:472–99.
12. Juel VC, Massey JM. Myasthenia gravis. Orphanet J Rare Dis 2007;2:44.
13. Pasnoor M, Wolfe GI, Nations S, et al. Clinical findings in MuSK-antibody positive myasthenia gravis: a U.S. experience. Muscle Nerve 2010;41:370–4.
14. Guptill JT, Sanders DB, Evoli A. Anti-MuSK antibody myasthenia gravis: clinical findings and response to treatment in two large cohorts. Muscle Nerve 2011;44:36–40.

15. Gwathmey KG, Burns TM. Myasthenia gravis. Semin Neurol 2015;35:327–39.
16. Gilhus NE. Myasthenia gravis. N Engl J Med 2016;375:2570–81.
17. Jani-Acsadi A, Lisak RP. Myasthenic crisis: guidelines for prevention and treatment. J Neurol Sci 2007;261:127–33.
18. Elsheikh B, Arnold WD, Gharibshahi S, et al. Correlation of single-breath count test and neck flexor muscle strength with spirometry in myasthenia gravis. Muscle Nerve 2016;53:134–6.
19. Thieben MJ, Blacker DJ, Liu PY, et al. Pulmonary function tests and blood gases in worsening myasthenia gravis. Muscle Nerve 2005;32:664–7.
20. Bhanushali MJ, Wuu J, Benatar M. Treatment of ocular symptoms in myasthenia gravis. Neurology 2008;71:1335–41.
21. Benatar M, McDermott MP, Sanders DB, et al. Efficacy of prednisone for the treatment of ocular myasthenia (EPITOME): a randomized, controlled trial. Muscle Nerve 2016;53:363–9.
22. Marx A, Wilisch A, Schultz A, et al. Pathogenesis of myasthenia gravis. Virchows Arch 1997;430:355–64.
23. Lauriola L, Ranelletti F, Maggiano N, et al. Thymus changes in anti-MuSK-positive and -negative myasthenia gravis. Neurology 2005;64:536–8.
24. Wolfe GI, Kaminski HJ, Aban IB, et al. Randomized trial of thymectomy in myasthenia gravis. N Engl J Med 2016;375:511–22.
25. Sanders DB, Burns TM, Cutter GR, et al. Does change in acetylcholine receptor antibody level correlate with clinical change in myasthenia gravis? Muscle Nerve 2014;49:483–6.
26. Leite MI, Strobel P, Jones M, et al. Fewer thymic changes in MuSK antibody-positive than in MuSK antibody-negative MG. Ann Neurol 2005;57:444–8.
27. Evoli A, Padua L. Diagnosis and therapy of myasthenia gravis with antibodies to muscle-specific kinase. Autoimmun Rev 2013;12:931 5.
28. Rodriguez M, Gomez MR, Howard FM Jr, et al. Myasthenia gravis in children: long-term follow-up. Ann Neurol 1983;13:504–10.
29. Tandan R, Hehir MK 2nd, Waheed W, et al. Rituximab treatment of myasthenia gravis: a systematic review. Muscle Nerve 2017;56(2):185–96.
30. Gasperi C, Melms A, Schoser B, et al. Anti-agrin autoantibodies in myasthenia gravis. Neurology 2014;82:1976–83.
31. Zhang B, Tzartos JS, Belimezi M, et al. Autoantibodies to lipoprotein-related protein 4 in patients with double-seronegative myasthenia gravis. Arch Neurol 2012;69:445–51.
32. Gallardo E, Martinez-Hernandez E, Titulaer MJ, et al. Cortactin autoantibodies in myasthenia gravis. Autoimmun Rev 2014;13:1003–7.
33. Zisimopoulou P, Evangelakou P, Tzartos J, et al. A comprehensive analysis of the epidemiology and clinical characteristics of anti-LRP4 in myasthenia gravis. J Autoimmun 2014;52:139–45.
34. Meriggioli MN, Sanders DB. Advances in the diagnosis of neuromuscular junction disorders. Am J Phys Med Rehabil 2005;84:627–38.
35. Rodriguez Cruz PM, Huda S, Lopez-Ruiz P, et al. Use of cell-based assays in myasthenia gravis and other antibody-mediated diseases. Exp Neurol 2015;270:66–71.
36. Rodriguez Cruz PM, Al-Hajjar M, Huda S, et al. Clinical features and diagnostic usefulness of antibodies to clustered acetylcholine receptors in the diagnosis of seronegative myasthenia gravis. JAMA Neurol 2015;72:642–9.

37. Skeie GO, Mygland A, Treves S, et al. Ryanodine receptor antibodies in myasthenia gravis: epitope mapping and effect on calcium release in vitro. Muscle Nerve 2003;27:81–9.
38. Romi F, Aarli JA, Gilhus NE. Myasthenia gravis patients with ryanodine receptor antibodies have distinctive clinical features. Eur J Neurol 2007;14:617–20.
39. Millichap JG, Dodge PR. Diagnosis and treatment of myasthenia gravis in infancy, childhood, and adolescence: a study of 51 patients. Neurology 1960;10: 1007–14.
40. Andrews PI. Autoimmune myasthenia gravis in childhood. Semin Neurol 2004;24: 101–10.
41. Evoli A, Batocchi AP, Bartoccioni E, et al. Juvenile myasthenia gravis with prepubertal onset. Neuromuscul Disord 1998;8:561–7.
42. Haliloglu G, Anlar B, Aysun S, et al. Gender prevalence in childhood multiple sclerosis and myasthenia gravis. J Child Neurol 2002;17:390–2.
43. Mittal MK, Barohn RJ, Pasnoor M, et al. Ocular myasthenia gravis in an academic neuro-ophthalmology clinic: clinical features and therapeutic response. J Clin Neuromuscul Dis 2011;13(1):46–52.
44. Castro D, Derisavifard S, Anderson M, et al. Juvenile myasthenia gravis: a twenty-year experience. J Clin Neuromuscul Dis 2013;14:95–102.
45. Pineles SL, Avery RA, Moss HE, et al. Visual and systemic outcomes in pediatric ocular myasthenia gravis. Am J Ophthalmol 2010;150:453–9.e3.
46. Ashraf VV, Taly AB, Veerendrakumar M, et al. Myasthenia gravis in children: a longitudinal study. Acta Neurol Scand 2006;114:119–23.
47. Hoff JM, Daltveit AK, Gilhus NE. Myasthenia gravis in pregnancy and birth: identifying risk factors, optimising care. Eur J Neurol 2007;14:38–43.
48. Silvestri NJ, Wolfe GI. Treatment-refractory myasthenia gravis. J Clin Neuromuscul Dis 2014;15:167–78.
49. Sanders DB, Wolfe GI, Benatar M, et al. International consensus guidance for management of myasthenia gravis: executive summary. Neurology 2016;87: 419–25.
50. Zebardast N, Patwa HS, Novella SP, et al. Rituximab in the management of refractory myasthenia gravis. Muscle Nerve 2010;41:375–8.
51. Silvestri NJ, Wolfe GI. Rituximab in treatment-refractory myasthenia gravis. JAMA Neurol 2017;74:21–3.
52. Gajdos P, Chevret S, Clair B, et al. Clinical trial of plasma exchange and high-dose intravenous immunoglobulin in myasthenia gravis. Myasthenia gravis clinical study group. Ann Neurol 1997;41:789–96.
53. Barth D, Nabavi Nouri M, Ng E, et al. Comparison of IVIg and PLEX in patients with myasthenia gravis. Neurology 2011;76:2017–23.
54. Carr AS, Hoeritzauer AI, Kee R, et al. Acute neuromuscular respiratory failure: a population-based study of aetiology and outcome in Northern Ireland. Postgrad Med J 2014;90:201–4.
55. Jaretzki A 3rd, Barohn RJ, Ernstoff RM, et al. Myasthenia gravis: recommendations for clinical research standards. Task Force of the Medical Scientific Advisory Board of the Myasthenia Gravis Foundation of America. Neurology 2000;55: 16–23.
56. Grob D. Course and management of myasthenia gravis. J Am Med Assoc 1953; 153:529–32.
57. Grob D. Myasthenia gravis: current status of pathogenesis, clinical manifestations, and management. J Chronic Dis 1958;8:536–66.

Diagnosis of Myasthenia Gravis

Mamatha Pasnoor, MD*, Mazen M. Dimachkie, MD,
Constantine Farmakidis, MD, Richard J. Barohn, MD

KEYWORDS

- Myasthenia gravis • Edrophonium test • Repetitive nerve stimulation
- Single-fiber electromyography • Acetylcholine receptor–binding autoantibodies
- Muscle-specific tyrosine kinase (MuSK)
- Low-density lipoprotein receptor–related protein 4 (LRP4) • Agrin

KEY POINTS

- Edrophonium testing is rarely used to confirm due to logistical barriers as atropine has to be kept in the clinic and this needs a crash cart and code team to be available.
- Autoantibodies to acetylcholine receptor binding are highly sensitivity and specific in generalized myasthenia gravis (MG).
- Slow repetitive nerve stimulation is a helpful tool to document an impaired safety factor of neuromuscular transmission in MG.
- Single-fiber electromyography is tedious and has the highest sensitivity in both generalized and ocular MG, particularly in weak muscles.

Myasthenia gravis (MG) diagnosis depends on clinical symptoms, examination findings, and the following diagnostic testing. In most instances the clinician makes the diagnosis of MG based on the neurologic history and examination findings, and the diagnostic tests are usually performed to confirm the clinical diagnosis.

Disclosure Statement: Drs M. Pasnoor and C. Farmakidis have nothing to disclose. Dr M.M. Dimachkie is on the speaker's bureau or is a consultant for Alnylam, Baxalta, Catalyst, CSL-Behring, Mallinckrodt, Novartis NuFactor, and Terumo. He has also received grants from Alexion, Biomarin, Catalyst, CSL Behring, FDA/OPD, GSK, Grifols, MDA, NIH, Novartis, Orphazyme, Sanofi, and TMA. Dr R.J. Barohn is a consultant for NuFactor and is on the advisory board for Novartis. He has received an honorarium from Option Care and PlatformQ Health Education. He has received research grants from NIH, FDA/OOPD, NINDS, Novartis, Sanofi/Genzyme, Biomarin, IONIS, Teva, Cytokinetics, Eli Lilly, PCORI, ALSA, and PTC. This work was supported by a CTSA grant from NCATS awarded to the University of Kansas for Frontiers: University of Kansas Clinical and Translational Science Institute (# UL1TR002366) The contents are solely the responsibility of the authors and do not necessarily represent the official views of the NIH or NCATS.
Department of Neurology, University of Kansas Medical Center, 3901 Rainbow Boulevard, Mail Stop 2012, Kansas City, KS 66160, USA
* Corresponding author:
E-mail address: mpasnoor@kumc.edu

Neurol Clin 36 (2018) 261–274
https://doi.org/10.1016/j.ncl.2018.01.010
0733-8619/18/© 2018 Elsevier Inc. All rights reserved.

neurologic.theclinics.com

ICE PACK TEST

This test is commonly performed by ophthalmologists and generally thought to have good sensitivity and specificity, however, more subject to false-positive and false-negative results than the edrophonium chloride test. This test is often used in cases whereby patients are either old or medically unstable for the edrophonium test or if edrophonium testing is not available.

Method: A cold ice pack, disposable glove, or specimen filled with ice is applied to the ptotic eyes for 1 to 2 minutes. Improvement of ptosis shortly after application of ice indicates a positive result.

A cooler temperature inhibits acetylcholinesterase enzyme activity,[1] leading to a decreased breakdown of released acetylcholine in the neuromuscular junction (NMJ), thus, improving NMJ transmission.

COGAN LID TWITCH TEST

This test consists of a brief overshoot twitch of lid retraction following sudden return of the eyes to the primary position after a period of downgaze.[2] The lid will briefly twitch upward then settle back to its previous position. This sign is used to evaluate MG; however, it is not diagnostic for this and may be seen in other conditions. One study by Singman and colleagues[3] showed a sensitivity of 75% and a specificity of 99% of the Cogan lid twitch in evaluating MG.

EDROPHONIUM CHLORIDE (ENLON) TEST

Edrophonium chloride is a short-acting, reversible acetylcholinesterase inhibitor. It inhibits the breakdown of acetylcholine, which is a neurotransmitter that is released at the synaptic junction, thus, increasing the availability of acetylcholine at the NMJ leading to increased binding of acetylcholine to postsynaptic receptors, causing an alteration in the ion channels; this leads to generation of the action potential. Edrophonium testing was introduced in the 1950s. Before that, diagnostic testing for MG was done with physostigmine and neostigmine (prostigmine), both introduced by Mary Walker.[4,5]

Edrophonium testing is a useful diagnostic test for myasthenia gravis; however, this cannot be used for adjusting the medical treatment. An objective way to measure weakness should be present before considering this testing, and this is usually ptosis. A response of ocular movement can also be seen; but it is difficult to determine if the test is positive unless diplopia reduces extremely, which is infrequent. Therefore, ptosis is the best sign to measure at the bedside.

The edrophonium test is a simple test that can be performed easily in the outpatient setting and does not need to be done in the hospital setting. The intravenous (IV) administration of up to 10 mg of edrophonium chloride is a diagnostic test in the evaluation of potential patients with MG. The details of the testing are presented in **Box 1**. It is not used as frequently now with the advent of antibody testing. The edrophonium test can have several pitfalls. The most common mistake is that the physician performing the test does not have an objective parameter to measure before and after edrophonium administration. As noted earlier, the most useful parameter is the degree of ptosis in each eye. The palpebral fissure should be measured before the drug is administered. The best indication of a positive test is a significant increase in the palpebral fissure aperture or the opening of a completely ptotic eye (**Figs. 1** and **2**). If no ptosis is present, the edrophonium test may be difficult to interpret even in clear-cut cases of MG. If patients have a

Box 1
Edrophonium testing: method

1. Patients are instructed not to take certain medications including pyridostigmine bromide for at least 12 hours before the testing.

2. Identify the objective parameter that you can test, for example, ptosis.

3. Baseline measurements of the objective parameter are obtained; for example, for ptosis, measure the palpebral fissure length between the two eyelids in the center with patients looking straight ahead.

4. An IV needle is placed in the arm.

5. Edrophonium (10 mg/mL) is taken into a 1-mL tuberculin syringe, and 0.2 mL is injected initially. Wait for 30 to 60 seconds; if there are no side effects (fasciculations, sweating, nausea), the rest of the 0.8 mL is injected. Another method used by some physicians includes injecting 0.2 mL, wait for 5 minutes, and then give 0.3 mL; after 5 minutes, if there are no side effects, give the rest of the 0.5 mL.

6. Blood pressure and heart rate have to be monitored closely every 2 minutes during and for 10 minutes after the procedure.

7. Measurements of the objective parameter identified and measured at the baseline are repeated immediately after the injection.

severe restriction of extraocular movement and edrophonium dramatically improves the motility, the test is considered positive. However, subjective diplopia may not resolve unless edrophonium produces orthophoria in the eyes, which is rare. Measurements by an ophthalmologist before and after administration of edrophonium might be a useful measure in mild cases of diplopia. Significant improvement in dysarthria or in swallowing is another indication of a positive edrophonium test. A mild improvement in limb strength or subjective well-being is not sufficient to claim a positive test. In addition, a positive edrophonium test is not specific because transient subjective improvement is reported in other neurologic disorders, such as motor neuron disease and peripheral neuropathy.[6]

Serious side effects include slow heart rate, chest pain, weak pulse, increased sweating, dizziness, weak or shallow breathing, seizures, and trouble swallowing. Less serious side effects include watery eyes, vision problems, mild nausea, vomiting, diarrhea, stomach pain, weakness, or muscle twitching. When either side effects or a positive response are obtained, no further edrophonium should be given. Atropine is kept on hand for significant bradycardia; however, in the authors' experience, it is rarely if ever needed.

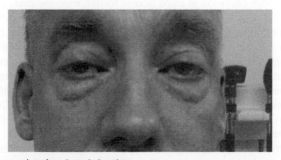

Fig. 1. Ptosis before edrophonium injection.

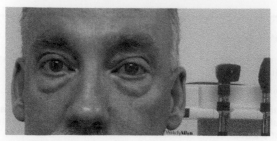

Fig. 2. Improvement in ptosis after edrophonium injection.

Edrophonium used to be supplied by a manufacturer that called the drug Tensilon; however, now there is a new manufacturer of the drug who uses the trade name Enlon.

If patients have ptosis, it is critical that the palpebral fissure aperture is measured and its size recorded before and after edrophonium administration. In patients with less objective findings that do not permit easy measurement, edrophonium should probably not be given in the first place. Thus, a placebo injection is rarely necessary.

In infants and younger children who are uncooperative and difficult to monitor over brief time periods, longer-acting neostigmine may be preferred. The intramuscular dose is 0.15 mg/kg, whereas the IV dose is 0.05 mg/kg.[7] IV use can be hazardous because of severe muscarinic side effects.[8] A positive response is generally evident by 15 minutes and is most obvious after 30 minutes. As with adults, atropine is kept on hand for significant bradycardia; however, in the authors' experience, it is rarely if ever needed.

In general, the authors think the edrophonium test is still useful in the diagnosis of MG. However, it is rarely performed now because of hospital restrictions and barriers imposed on allowing physicians to do the test in the outpatient setting. Thus, young neurologists rarely learn how to perform the test during training. The authors think that learning how to perform the edrophonium test should be part of the neurologist training. For more information about this test, the reader is referred to Mohammed Al-Haidar and colleagues' article, "Ocular Myasthenia Gravis," in this issue.

ANTIBODY TESTING
Anti–Acetylcholine Receptor Antibodies

Finding elevated acetylcholine receptor (AChR) antibody levels in the serum of patients with suspected MG is the most specific diagnostic test.

AChR-antibody levels are not elevated in all patients with MG. The assay is most helpful in adult generalized MG; it is positive in 85% of such patients.[9–12] Patients with ocular MG, however, have a measurable AChR antibody in only 50% of cases.[13] Seronegativity is more common in pure ocular forms, mild disease, and remission.[14] Because congenital myasthenic syndromes and seronegative autoimmune MG present in early childhood, differentiating these disorders when the family history is negative is often difficult.[7] Fluctuating weakness or disease severity and good responses to immunotherapy favor an autoimmune basis.[15] The availability of genetic testing for Congenital Myasthenic Syndrome (CMS) has also improved diagnostic yield, though sensitivity remains moderate. The most common CMS mutations are in the Choline receptor epsilon subunit gene for AChR protein (CHRNE), RAPSN (codes for rapsyn protein) and Collagen like tail subunit of asymmetric acetylcholinesterase (ColQ) encoding genes.

The most common AChR-antibody test is the binding radioimmunoassay using bungarotoxin, measured in nanomoles per liter. The upper limit of normal varies among reference laboratories (usually between 0.03 and 0.5 nmol/L).[16] Other assays that block bungarotoxin binding to AChR (blocking assay) or that reduce the density of AChR on cultured human myotubes (modulating antibody assay) are also commercially available.[17] These additional assays may be useful in patients with suspected MG who test negative with the standard binding assay,[17] but do not add significantly to the diagnostic sensitivity. Some laboratories offer all 3 (binding, blocking, and modulating) antibodies as one serologic test. High titers of modulating antibody titers have been associated with more frequency of thymoma but these are not specific and do not replace the need for chest computerized axial tomography imaging. Recently, low-affinity AChR antibodies against rapsyn-clustered AChR were seen in 66% of patients who were otherwise seronegative. These antibodies were mainly immunoglobulin G1 (IgG1) antibodies that can activate complement C3b deposition.[18,19]

AChR-antibody titers correlate poorly with MG severity.[20] Although the titer often decreases as the clinical condition improves, antibody titers in general do not guide therapeutic decisions. Indeed, patients with MG in clinical remission may still have elevated titers, but this is not an indication to continue immunosuppressive therapy.

Anti–Muscle-Specific Receptor Tyrosine Kinase Antibodies

Since 2001, IgG from 40% to 70% of seronegative generalized patients has been found to bind to the extracellular domain of muscle-specific receptor tyrosine kinase (MuSK)[21–23] or 7% of all generalized MG cases. It has been hypothesized that anti-MuSK antibodies impede agrin-mediated clustering of AChR and disrupt normal postsynaptic architecture.[24] Marked female predominance with a mean age of onset in the fourth decade has been typical.[23,25] The earliest reported onset of anti-MuSK MG is 2 years old.[26] Three main patterns of anti-MuSK MG have been observed; one of them is clinically indistinguishable from anti-AChR generalized MG. The other two patterns are severe oculobulbar weakness and prominent neck, shoulder, and respiratory involvement largely sparing ocular musculature. Midline tongue atrophy is a clue to the diagnosis of MuSK MG (**Fig. 3**). In these two phenotypic variants, limb strength is relatively intact.[23,27] Anti-MuSK antibodies are rarely seen in pure ocular MG.[28] MuSK MG is somewhat more refractory to conventional treatment when compared with AChR MG.[29] Testing for anti-MuSK antibodies should be considered in all patients with suspected MG who are AChR-antibody negative.

Striated Muscle Antibodies and Other Laboratory Studies

Antibodies to striated muscle in patients with MG were discovered before AChR-Ab. These antibodies can be directed against several muscle proteins, including myosin,

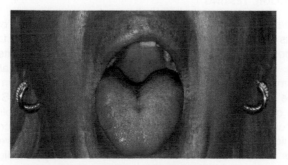

Fig. 3. Midline tongue atrophy in a patient with MuSK MG.

actin, alpha-actinin, titin, and ryanodine receptor (RyR). It is generally thought that if antistriated muscle antibodies are present in patients with MG, they should raise suspicion for thymoma, as they are reported in up to 84% of patients with thymoma.[30] However, these antibodies may be found in patients without thymoma and in patients with thymoma, who do not have MG.[31,32] The absence of antistriated antibodies also does not rule out thymoma. Antititin and RyR antibodies have been observed as a marker for more severe disease in patients with MG presenting after 40 years of age.[31] Thyroid function tests are routinely obtained at the time of the initial evaluation, as thyroid disease often coexists with MG.[33]

Lipoprotein-Related Protein 4

Low-density lipoprotein-related protein 4 (LRP4) is a recently identified antibody. LRP4 interacts with agrin, and this activates MuSK and promotes the clustering of the AChR and their stabilization at the NMJ. Anti-LRP4 antibodies are found in approximately 9.2% (range 2%–50%) of patients with MG who are negative for both anti-AChR and anti-MuSK antibodies.[34] LRP4 antibody testing has recently become commercially available. A study investigating the clinical profile of LRP4/agrin antibody-positive MG will also evaluate the sensitivity and specificity of these autoantibodies.

In some patients in whom AChR and MuSK antibodies are not detectable by conventional assays, circulating antibodies can be detected by the binding of clustered AChRs in a cell-based assay.[35] Anti-Kv1.4 antibodies that target α-subunits (Kv 1.4) of the voltage-gated potassium channels (VGKC) have been reported in 12% to 28% of Japanese patients with MG[36,37] and also found in mild or predominantly ocular MG in a Caucasian cohort.[37] These antibodies present in MG without clinical or electrical neuromyotonia, suggesting that the targeted antigen may not be a neuronal VGKC and perhaps the VGKC on muscle fibers.

Rapsyn is an intracellular end-plate protein that is necessary for the clustering of AChRs at the postsynaptic folds of the NMJ.[38] Antirapsyn antibodies have been found in patients with MG, most commonly in the thymomatous MG, but have also been found in patients with other autoimmune diseases. Antibodies to end-plate acetylcholinesterase have also been reported in patients with MG; but the pathogenic role of these antibodies is questionable, as they are present in other autoimmune diseases and healthy controls. For more discussion on autoantibodies in MG, the reader is referred to Michael H. Rivner and colleagues' article, "MuSK and Myasthenia Gravis due to Other Autoantibodies," in this issue.

ELECTROPHYSIOLOGIC TESTING

Repetitive stimulation: The classic electrophysiologic demonstration of an NMJ transmission defect is the documentation of a decremental response of the compound muscle action potential (CMAP) to slow (2–3 Hz) motor repetitive nerve stimulation (RNS)[39] (**Fig. 4**). Although decrement on slow-frequency RNS is also seen in the Lambert-Eaton myasthenic syndrome (LEMS), the typical pattern in this disease is marked increase (doubling) of the CMAP amplitude with fast RNS rates of 30 to 50 Hz, which is quite painful (**Fig. 5**). A 100 or greater CMAP amplitude increment following 10 seconds of maximal exercise is a less noxious way of confirming LEMS electrophysiologically. For a more detailed discussion on LEMS, the reader is referred to Vita G. Kesner and colleagues' article, "Lambert-Eaton Myasthenic Syndrome," in this issue.

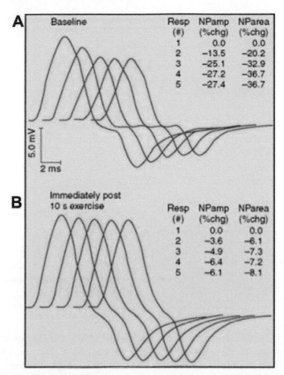

Fig. 4. Typical pattern of decrement in a patient with MG. Repetitive stimulation of the ulnar nerve at 3 Hz, record adductor digiti minimi. (A) Baseline, abnormal amplitude decrement of 27%. (B) Immediately after 10 seconds of exercise, the decrement has resolved, demonstrating repair. NPamp, negative peak amplitude; NParea, negative peak area; Resp, response. (*Adapted from* Silvestri NJ, Barohn RJ, Wolfe GI. Acquired disorders of neuromuscular junction. In: Swaiman KF, editor. Swaiman's pediatric neurology, principles and practice. 6th edition. Philadelphia: Elsevier; 2017; with permission.)

The decrement on slow-frequency RNS is due to failure of some muscle fibers to reach the threshold and contract when successive volleys of ACh vesicles are released at the NMJ. Failure to reach the threshold end-plate potential (EPP) to achieve muscle contraction is called blocking. The percent decrease in amplitude and area is calculated between the first CMAP produced by a train of stimuli and each successive one. In most laboratories, 5 responses are obtained at 2 or 3 Hz, and the maximal percent decrement can be measured at the fourth or fifth response. A decrement of greater than 10% is considered a positive RNS study. The 10% level takes into account potential technical results so that amplitude changes less than this are not considered necessarily pathologic. However, there really should be no decrement in healthy individuals. Lower cutoff values for pathologic decrement have been suggested[40]; but caution should be exerted not to extrapolate data to other laboratories without further local validation, as this test is fraught with significant technical challenges. Some laboratories prefer 9 responses; when this is done, a slight return of the CMAP amplitude can be seen after 4 or 5 CMAPs in MG. Finally, and in addition to the diagnostic value, higher jitter and decrement values were associated with more severe MG disease.[41]

In some patients, a decremental response can be demonstrated at baseline. However, often a brief period of exercise (usually 1 minute) is required to fatigue the NMJ so

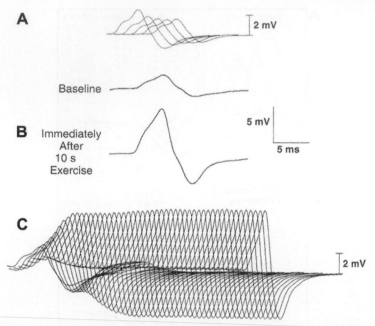

Fig. 5. The triad of electrodiagnostic abnormalities in LEMS. (*A*) Decremental response on low-frequency stimulation. (*B*) Low-amplitude baseline CMAP that increases in amplitude and area by more than 100% after brief exercise or with (*C*) high-frequency repetitive stimulation for 1 second. (*Adapted from* Silvestri NJ, Barohn RJ, Wolfe GI. Acquired disorders of neuromuscular junction. In: Swaiman KF, editor. Swaiman's pediatric neurology, principles and practice. 6th edition. Philadelphia: Elsevier; 2017; with permission.)

that the decrement can be observed. This phenomenon of postexercise exhaustion (PEE) usually occurs at 2 to 4 minutes after exercise. In addition, repair or an improvement in the decrement can sometimes be observed immediately (within seconds) after brief exercise (postexercise facilitation) (**Fig. 6**).

RNS is typically first recorded in a distal thenar or hypothenar muscle after stimulating the median or ulnar nerve, respectively, for generalized MG. For ocular MG, typically a orbicularis oculi or nasalis response is recorded while stimulating the facial nerve. If no decrement is observed, RNS can be performed on a proximal limb muscle (ie, trapezius, face, deltoid, biceps). An arm board is used to immobilize the hand muscles. False-positive results are more of a problem in proximal limb muscles because of motion artifact. In stimulating proximal nerves, it is helpful to have another individual assisting the electromyographer to hold the patients' shoulders down and head still.

As with the edrophonium test, RNS does not have to be performed on every patient with MG if the diagnosis is certain based on clinical findings and a positive AChR antibody (**Box 2**).

Because RNS is a reflection of the integrity of NMJ transmission, a decrement is more often observed in clinically weak muscles. Thus, even if patients have generalized MG, if there is only facial and proximal limb weakness, a decrement in a hand muscle is unlikely. In patients with pure ocular MG, a decrement may not be present in the orbicularis oculi unless that muscle is weak on examination.

A decremental response is more likely present in a proximal muscle than in a distal muscle. In the series by Stalberg and Sanders,[42] a decrement in a distal muscle was

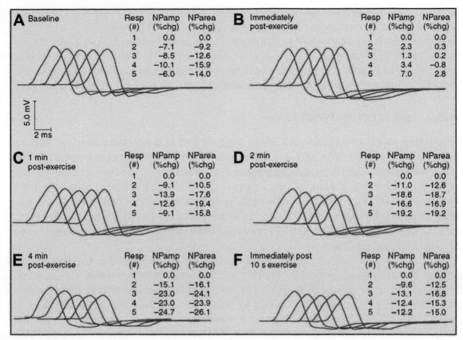

Fig. 6. Repetitive stimulation of the ulnar nerve at 3 Hz, record adductor digiti minimi. (*A*) At baseline there is only a borderline decrement at response 4. (*B–E*) After exercise, a 12% to 13% decrement develops immediately (*B*) and 1 minute (*C*) after exercise; this worsens at 2 and 4 minutes (*D*, *E*), demonstrating PEE. (*F*) After 10 seconds of brief exercise, the decrement improves. NPamp, negative peak amplitude; NParea, negative peak area; Resp, response. (*Adapted from* Silvestri NJ, Barohn RJ, Wolfe GI. Acquired disorders of neuromuscular junction. In: Swaiman KF, editor. Swaiman's pediatric neurology, principles and practice. 6th edition. Philadelphia: Elsevier; 2017; with permission.)

reported in 38% of patients, whereas a decrement in proximal muscles occurred in 64%. Similar findings have been described by other investigators.[11,43] In ocular MG, decrements are less common, occurring in 20% to 50% of patients.[42,44] Facial muscle RNS should be included when clinical suspicion for anti-MuSK myasthenia exists, as

---

Box 2
Protocol for repetitive nerve stimulation of the ulnar nerve recording over the adductor digiti minimi

- Apply electrodes and immobilize the hand.

- Obtain a normal baseline CMAP, and increase to supramaximal intensity.

- If there is as small CMAP amplitude at the baseline, screen for LEMS before doing RNS.

- After establishing a stable baseline CMAP, give 5 stimuli at 3 Hz.

- If there is no decrement, exercise the hand by having patients abduct the fingers for 1 minute. Repeat RNS immediately after exercise and at 1, 2, 4, and 6 minutes after exercise.

- If there is a decrement after exercise (PEE), briefly exercise the muscle again for 10 seconds and repeat RNS at 3 Hz. If the decrement now improves, this indicates repair.

- A CMAP amplitude decrement of greater than 10% from baseline is considered abnormal.

facial muscles are much more prominently involved in this group.[27] RNS at faster rates (ie, 20 or 50 Hz) is performed when there is concern about LEMS.

Although RNS is a useful test to diagnose MG, in new patients diagnosed with positive AChR antibodies, there is probably no need to do the RNS to find the decremental response. RNS is probably most useful in patients first presenting with MG symptoms and AChR-antibody results are unavailable and in AchR-antibody–negative patients.

SINGLE-FIBER ELECTROMYOGRAPHY

Single-fiber electromyography (SFEMG) (**Figs. 7** and **8**) was established by Stalberg and Eskedt[45] in the 1960s and is a more sensitive measure of neuromuscular transmission than RNS, and it can be considered if other testing is negative and clinical suspicion is high for MG.[46] When a motor axon is depolarized, the action potentials travel distally and excite the muscle fibers more or less at the same time. In MG, the time required for the EPP at the NMJ to reach the threshold is extremely variable. The measurement of this variability in the EPP increase time between 2 fibers of the same motor unit is known as jitter.

Most of the electromyography (EMG) machines have software to perform and analyze the SFEMG examination. There are 2 methods to perform this. One is stimulated and the other is volitional effort. The volitional is most commonly used by most physicians. Usually patients are asked to hold their anticholinesterase inhibitors for 24 hours before the study. Orbicularis oris, extensor digitorum communis, or frontalis are the most common muscles tested. A single-fiber needle or concentric needle electrode inserted into the muscle, and individual muscle fiber pairs are selectively identified and the EPPs recorded. The low-frequency filter and high-frequency filter settings can be adjusted to increase the selectivity of the recording. The low-frequency filter is set at 500 Hz and the high-frequency filter at 10 KHz for a single-fiber needle; for a concentric needle, the low-frequency filter is set at 1 KHz, usually to filter out EPPs of distant muscle fibers. The recorded potential should be greater than 200 μV in amplitude, and the increase time should be less than 300 microseconds. Twenty potential pairs are collected from the same muscle by 3 to 4 insertions. One hundred consecutive discharges are recorded from each pair. Patients are asked to maintain steady contraction for volitional SFEMG until 100 discharges are recorded from each pair. Stimulated SFEMG is useful for children, uncooperative patients, comatose patients, and those who have tremors. A fascicle of motor nerve is stimulated by using a monopolar needle electrode, and recording is made by SFEMG or a concentric

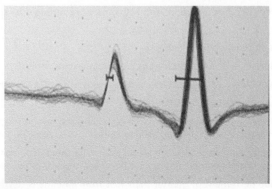

Fig. 7. Normal SFEMG.

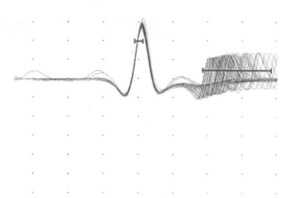

Fig. 8. Abnormal SFEMG.

needle electrode and recording is made by SFEMG or a concentric needle electrode. Stimulation is delivered at 2 to 10 Hz, and the stimulus intensity is adjusted accordingly.

The jitter value is the measurement of the variation of the interpotential interval between the triggered potential and the time-locked, second single muscle fiber potential; it is calculated as the mean consecutive difference in microseconds and is the most important piece of data obtained from SFEMG. Everyone, including healthy individuals, have some degree of jitter. Myasthenic patients have increased jitter values. The normal jitter values have been determined for many muscles in multicenter collaborative studies.[47] The study is considered abnormal if either the mean jitter value exceeds the upper limit of normal value or more than 10% of the pairs have increased jitter (more than 2 out of the 20 pairs). In addition, blocking occurs in myasthenic patients if a muscle fiber's EPP never reaches the threshold and depolarization does not occur. The frequency of blocking, expressed as a percentage, is also determined with SFEMG. In healthy individuals, the percentage of blocking is 0%.

SFEMG is the most sensitive test for MG in adults. It is abnormal in 94% of patients with generalized MG and 80% of patients with ocular MG.[11,48] However, SFEMG has several disadvantages. It is a tedious and lengthy study that requires considerable patient cooperation and is poorly tolerated by many people. The need to use nondisposable single-fiber electrodes was also a limitation; but there have been recent normative data for single-fiber studies with disposable concentric needles.[49] Stimulated SFEMG can be performed under sedation, requires less patient cooperation, and may be preferred in children, although it is still a lengthy procedure.[50] An abnormal SFEMG study is not specific for MG because increased jitter commonly occurs as a result of other neuromuscular diseases, including motor neuron disease, peripheral neuropathy, and many myopathies.[39] However, it is also true that if SFEMG is normal in a weak muscle, it almost completely excludes the diagnosis of myasthenia. Conventional needle EMG has limited diagnostic value in MG; however, short-duration, small-amplitude early recruited myopathic units can be seen in patients with MuSK MG[51] and in severe MG cases.

A comparison made between the diagnostic yield of repetitive stimulation, antibody titers, and SFEMG showed that SFEMG was highly sensitive (99%), followed by the AChR antibody; the least sensitive was repetitive stimulation (76%), if the proximal muscles were tested.[52] Repetitive stimulation was technically difficult, and a mild decremental response was well recognized in motor neuron disease and peripheral neuropathies.[53] In MG, a decremental response was less pronounced in the distal muscles than the proximal muscles. AChR antibody is detected in only 50% of patients with ocular MG and 85% of patients with generalized MG.[54] A portion of these patients have MuSK or recently identified LRP4 antibodies.

REFERENCES

1. Movaghar M, Slavin ML. Effect of local heat versus ice on blepharoptosis resulting from ocular myasthenia. Ophthalmology 2000;107:2209–14.
2. Cogan DG. Myasthenia gravis: a review of the disease and a description of lid twitch as a characteristic sign. Arch Ophthalmol 1965;74:217–21.
3. Singman EL, Matta NS, Silbert DI. Use of the Cogan lid twitch to identify myasthenia gravis. J Neuroophthalmol 2011;31(3):239–40.
4. Walker MB. Treatment of myasthenia gravis with physostigmine. Lancet 1934; 223:1200–1.
5. Walker M. The treatment of myasthenia gravis. Med press 1946;216:81–4.
6. Oh SJ, Cho HK. Edrophonium responsiveness not necessarily diagnostic of myasthenia gravis. Muscle Nerve 1990;13:187–91.
7. Andrews PI. Autoimmune myasthenia gravis in childhood. Semin Neurol 2004;24: 101–10.
8. Wolfe GI, Barohn RJ, Galetta SL. Drugs for the diagnosis and treatment of myasthenia gravis. In: Zimmerman T, Kooner K, Sharir M, et al, editors. Textbook of Ocular Pharmacology. Philadelphia: Lippincott-Raven Press; 1997. p. 837–48.
9. Drachman DB. Myasthenia gravis. N Engl J Med 1994;330:1797–810.
10. Lindstrom JM, Seybold ME, Lennon VA, et al. Antibody to acetylcholine-receptor in myasthenia-gravis - prevalence, clinical correlates, and diagnostic value. Neurology 1976;26:1054–9.
11. Oh SJ, Kim DE, Kuruoglu R, et al. Diagnostic sensitivity of the laboratory tests in myasthenia gravis. Muscle Nerve 1992;15:720–4.
12. Vincent A, Newsom-Davis J. Acetylcholine receptor antibody as a diagnostic test for myasthenia gravis: results in 153 validated cases and 2967 diagnostic assays. J Neurol Neurosurg Psychiatry 1985;48:1246–52.
13. Provenzano C, Marino M, Scuderi F, et al. Anti-acetylcholinesterase antibodies associate with ocular myasthenia gravis. J Neuroimmunol 2010;218(1–2):102–6.
14. Afifi AK, Bell WE. Tests for juvenile myasthenia gravis: comparative diagnostic yield and prediction of outcome. J Child Neurol 1993;8:403–11.
15. Anlar B, Ozdirim E, Renda Y, et al. Myasthenia gravis in childhood. Acta Paediatr 1996;85:838–42.
16. Lennon VA. Myasthenia gravis - diagnosis by assay of serum antibodies. Mayo Clin Proc 1982;57:723–4.
17. Howard FM Jr, Lennon VA, Finley J, et al. Clinical correlations of antibodies that bind, block, or modulate human acetylcholine receptors in myasthenia gravis. Ann N Y Acad Sci 1987;505:526–38.
18. Leite MI, Jacob S, Viegas S, et al. IgG1 antibodies to acetylcholine receptors in 'seronegative' myasthenia gravis. Brain 2008;131:1940–52.
19. Vincent A, Leite MI, Farrugia ME, et al. Myasthenia gravis seronegative for acetylcholine receptor antibodies. Ann N Y Acad Sci 2008;1132:84–92.
20. Roses AD, Olanow CW, McAdams MW, et al. No direct correlation between serum antiacetylcholine receptor antibody levels and clinical state of individual patients with myasthenia gravis. Neurology 1981;31:220–4.

21. Hoch W, McConville J, Helms S, et al. Auto-antibodies to the receptor tyrosine kinase MuSK in patients with myasthenia gravis without acetylcholine receptor antibodies. Nat Med 2001;7:365–8.
22. McConville J, Farrugia ME, Beeson D, et al. Detection and characterization of MuSK antibodies in seronegative myasthenia gravis. Ann Neurol 2004;55:580–4.
23. Sanders DB, El-Salem K, Massey JM, et al. Clinical aspects of MuSK antibody positive seronegative MG. Neurology 2003;60:1978–80.
24. Jha S, Xu K, Maruta T, et al. Myasthenia gravis induced in mice by immunization with the recombinant extracellular domain of rat muscle-specific kinase (MuSK). J Neuroimmunol 2006;175:107–17.
25. Evoli A, Tonali PA, Padua L, et al. Clinical correlates with anti-MuSK antibodies in generalized seronegative myasthenia gravis. Brain 2003;126:2304–11.
26. Murai H, Noda T, Himeno E, et al. Infantile onset myasthenia gravis with MuSK antibodies. Neurology 2006;67:174.
27. Muppidi S, Wolfe GI. Muscle-specific receptor tyrosine kinase antibody-positive and seronegative myasthenia gravis. Front Neurol Neurosci 2009;26:109–19.
28. Wolfe GI, Trivedi JR, Oh SJ. Clinical review of muscle-specific tyrosine kinase-antibody positive myasthenia gravis. J Clin Neuromuscul Dis 2007;8:217–24.
29. Pasnoor M, Wolfe GI, Nations S, et al. Clinical findings in MuSK-antibody positive myasthenia gravis: a U.S. experience. Muscle Nerve 2009;41(3):370–4.
30. Limburg PC, The TH, Hummeltappel E, et al. Anti-acetylcholine receptor antibodies in myasthenia-gravis. Part 1. Relation to clinical-parameters in 250 patients. J Neurol Sci 1983;58:357–70.
31. Romi F, Skeie GO, Aarli JA, et al. The severity of myasthenia gravis correlates with the serum concentration of titin and ryanodine receptor antibodies. Arch Neurol 2000;57:1596–600.
32. Cikes N, Momoi MY, Williams CL, et al. Striational autoantibodies: quantitative detection by enzyme immunoassay in myasthenia gravis, thymoma, and recipients of D-penicillamine or allogeneic bone marrow. Mayo Clin Proc 1988;63:474–81.
33. Meriggioli MN, Sanders DB. Autoimmune myasthenia gravis: emerging clinical and biological heterogeneity. Lancet Neurol 2009;8:475–90.
34. Zhang B, Tzartos JS, Belimezi M, et al. Autoantibodies to lipoprotein-related protein 4 in patients with double-seronegative myasthenia gravis. Arch Neurol 2012;69:445–51.
35. Vincent A, Waters P, Leite MI, et al. Antibodies identified by cell-based assays in myasthenia gravis and associated diseases. Ann N Y Acad Sci 2012;1274:92–8.
36. Suzuki S, Satoh T, Yasuoka H, et al. Novel autoantibodies to a voltage-gated potassium channel Kv1.4 in a severe form of myasthenia gravis. J Neuroimmunol 2005;170:141–9.
37. Romi F, Suzuki S, Suzuki N, et al. Anti-voltage-gated potassium channel Kv1.4 antibodies in myasthenia gravis. J Neurol 2012;259:1312–6.
38. Agius MA, Zhu S, Kirvan CA, et al. Rapsyn antibodies in myasthenia gravis. Ann N Y Acad Sci 1998;841:516–21.
39. Oh SJ. Electromyography: neuromuscular transmission studies. Baltimore (MD): Williams & Wilkins; 1988.
40. Abraham A, Alabdali M, Alsulaiman A, et al. Repetitive nerve stimulation cutoff values for the diagnosis of myasthenia gravis. Muscle Nerve 2017;55:166–70.
41. Abraham A, Breiner A, Barnett C, et al. Electrophysiological testing is correlated with myasthenia gravis severity. Muscle Nerve 2017;56:445–8.

42. Stalberg E, Sanders DB. Electrophysiologic testing of neuromuscular transmission. In: Stalberg E, Young RR, editors. Clinical neurophysiology. London: Butterworth; 1981. p. 88–116.
43. Vial C, Charles N, Chauplannaz G, et al. Myasthenia gravis in childhood and infancy. Usefulness of electrophysiologic studies. Arch Neurol 1991;48:847–9.
44. Evoli A, Tonali P, Bartoccioni E, et al. Ocular myasthenia: diagnostic and therapeutic problems. Acta Neurol Scand 1988;77:31–5.
45. Ekstedt J, Stålberg E. The effect of non-paralytic doses of D-tubocurarine on individual motor end-plates in man, studied with a new electrophysiological method. Electroencephalogr Clin Neurophysiol 1969;27(6):557–62.
46. Padua L, Stalberg E, LoMonaco M, et al. SFEMG in ocular myasthenia gravis diagnosis. Clin Neurophysiol 2000;111:1203–7.
47. Bromberg MB, Scott DM. Single fiber EMG reference values: reformatted in tabular form. AD HOC Committee of the AAEM Single Fiber Special Interest Group. Muscle Nerve 1994;17:820–1.
48. Sanders DB, Howard JF Jr. AAEE minimonograph #25: single-fiber electromyography in myasthenia gravis. Muscle Nerve 1986;9:809–19.
49. Stalberg EV, Sanders DB. Jitter recordings with concentric needle electrodes. Muscle Nerve 2009;40:331–9.
50. Jabre JF, Chirico-Post J, Weiner M. Stimulation SFEMG in myasthenia gravis. Muscle Nerve 1989;12:38–42.
51. Padua L, Tonali P, Aprile I, et al. Seronegative myasthenia gravis: comparison of neurophysiological picture in MuSK+ and MuSK- patients. Eur J Neurol 2006;13: 273–6.
52. Sanders DB, Stalberg EV. AAEM minimonograph #25: single-fiber electromyography. Muscle Nerve 1996;19:1069–83.
53. Farrugia ME, Jacob S, Sarrigiannis PG, et al. Correlating extent of neuromuscular instability with acetylcholine receptor antibodies. Muscle Nerve 2009;39:489–93.
54. Milone M, Monaco ML, Evoli A, et al. Ocular myasthenia: diagnostic value of single fibre EMG in the orbicularis oculi muscle. J Neurol Neurosurg Psychiatry 1993;56:720–1.

Nature and Action of Antibodies in Myasthenia Gravis

Robert L. Ruff, MD, PhD[a,b], Robert P. Lisak, MD, FRCP[c,d],*

KEYWORDS

- Acetylcholine esterases • Acetylcholine receptors • Autoantibodies • Complement
- Muscle specific kinase • Neuromuscular transmission • Sodium channels

KEY POINTS

- This article discusses the antibodies associated with immune-mediated myasthenia gravis and the pathologic action of these antibodies at the neuromuscular junctions of skeletal muscle.
- We explain how the pathologic antibodies act, and consider the physiology of neuromuscular transmission with emphasis on 4 features.
- We describe the structure of the neuromuscular junction and the roles of postsynaptic acetylcholine receptors and voltage-gated Na⁺ channels.
- We discuss the safety factor for neuromuscular transmission and how the safety factor is reduced in different forms of autoimmune myasthenia gravis.

ACETYLCHOLINE IS THE TRANSMITTER AT THE NEUROMUSCULAR JUNCTION

Acetylcholine (ACh) is stored in vesicles in the nerve terminal (**Fig. 1**).[1] ACh-containing vesicles are aligned near the ACh release sites or active zones where the vesicles will fuse with the presynaptic nerve terminal membrane.[1] Release sites are located opposite the clefts and between the tops of the secondary synaptic folds of the postsynaptic muscle membrane.[1–3] Transmitter release requires Ca^{2+} entry via P/Q-type Ca^{2+} channels.[4]

THE ROLE OF THE SYNAPTIC CLEFT

The space between the nerve terminal and the postsynaptic membrane, the synaptic cleft, is about 50 nm (see **Fig. 1**).[1] ACh diffuses across the synaptic cleft to activate

^a Department of Neurology, Case Western University School of Medicine, The Metro Health System, 2500 Metro Health Drive, Cleveland, OH 44109, USA; ^b Department of Neurosciences, Case Western Reserve University, Cleveland, OH, USA; ^c Department of Neurology, Wayne State University School of Medicine, 8D University Health Center, 4201 St Antoine, Detroit, MI 48201, USA; ^d Department of Biochemistry, Microbiology and Immunology, Wayne State University, Detroit, MI, USA
* Corresponding author. Department of Neurology, Wayne State University School of Medicine, 8D University Health Center, 4201 St Antoine, Detroit, MI 48201, USA.
E-mail address: rlisak@med.wayne.edu

Neurol Clin 36 (2018) 275–291
https://doi.org/10.1016/j.ncl.2018.01.001   **neurologic.theclinics.com**
0733-8619/18/© 2018 Elsevier Inc. All rights reserved.

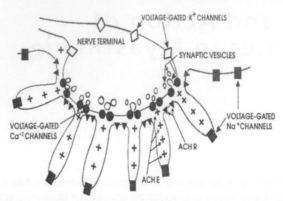

Fig. 1. Depiction of the neuromuscular junction. The nerve terminal is located above the secondary synaptic folds of the postsynaptic muscle membrane. The nerve terminal contains mitochondria, which produce the energy needed to synthesize acetylcholine (ACh) and package the ACh into synaptic vesicles. Synaptic vesicles can fuse with the nerve terminal membrane after an AP enters the nerve terminal. The nerve terminal contains voltage-gated K^+ channels ($\diamond$) and Ca^{2+} channels ($\bullet$). Active zones, where Ca^{2+} channels are concentrated and synaptic vesicles fuse with the presynaptic membrane, are precisely aligned above troughs between secondary synaptic folds of the postsynaptic membrane. Within the synaptic cleft, the extracellular matrix contains acetylcholine esterase (AChE) (+) that is bound to the basal lamina of the postsynaptic membrane. The secondary synaptic folds contain a high density of acetylcholine receptors (AChR) ($\blacktriangledown$) on the tops of the secondary folds close to the nerve terminal membrane and a high density of Na^+ channels at the bottom of the troughs of the secondary synaptic folds ($\blacksquare$).

ACh receptors (AChRs). Each synaptic vesicle releases about 10,000 ACh molecules into the synaptic cleft.[5] Adenosine triphosphate is also released from synaptic vesicles and the released adenosine triphosphate may modulate transmitter release of post-synaptic transmitter sensitivity.[6] An action potential (AP) in the nerve terminal stimulates between 50 and 300 synaptic vesicles to fuse (ie, the normal quantal content is between 50 and 300).[7] The diffusion of ACh across the synaptic cleft is very rapid owing to the small distance to be traversed and the high diffusion constant for ACh.[8] ACh esterase (AChE) in the basal lamina of the postsynaptic membrane and the synaptic cleft accelerates the disappearance of ACh from the synaptic cleft, as does diffusion of ACh out of the cleft.[9,10] Inactivation of AChE prolongs the duration of action of ACh on the postsynaptic membrane and slow the decay of the ACh-induced endplate current (EPC).[9] The concentration of AChE is approximately 3000 molecules/μm^2 of postsynaptic membrane.[9] AChRs have a concentration of about 15,000 to 20,000 molecules/μm^2 of postsynaptic membrane.[11] The concentration of AChE is great enough that most of the ACh entering a synaptic cleft is hydrolyzed to prevent AChRs from being activated more than once by nerve terminal released ACh.[12]

POSTSYNAPTIC MEMBRANE

The postsynaptic membrane is a complex collection of proteins that serve many purposes including the concentration and localization of 2 key elements, AChRs and voltage-gated skeletal muscle Na^+ channels, which convert the chemical signal from the motor neuron and ACh, into an electrical signal, the AP, that rapidly travels to the tendon ends of each muscle fiber. The AP triggers release of Ca^{2+} from intracellular stores, leading to muscle fiber contraction, a process called excitation contraction coupling.[13–15] The details of the cast and actions of the complex proteins that contribute to the concentration and localization of AChRs are summarized by Wu and colleagues.[16] AChR clustering at the apex of secondary synaptic folds are mediated via complex interactions of a plethora of proteins (**Fig. 2A**).[16] The important proteins include agrin, DOK7, low-density lipoprotein receptor-related protein 4 (LRP4), muscle-specific receptor tyrosine kinase (MuSK), and rapsyn (**Fig. 3**).[16,17] Rapsyn and DOK7 also contribute to AChR clustering.[16,18–21] Rapsyn is the molecular glue that links AChRs together in clusters.[19] Na^+ channel concentration at the endplate involves agrin, ankryn, and syntrophin.[22–27]

HOW SECONDARY SYNAPTIC FOLDS ELECTRICALLY COUPLE ACETYLCHOLINE RECEPTORS AND NA$^+$ CHANNELS

The postsynaptic membrane area is increased by folding into secondary synaptic clefts or folds (see **Figs. 1** and **2A**).[28–34] AChRs are concentrated at the tops of the secondary synaptic folds closest to the nerve terminal.[18,35] The interaction between ACh and the AChRs opens the AChR cation-specific channel producing the localized endplate depolarization (EPP) that depolarizes the endplate Na^+ channels triggering APs that travel from the neuromuscular junction to the tendon ends of the muscle fiber (see **Fig. 2A**).[1,28–34] The conductance of the AChR ion channel is about 40 to 60 pS and the current flowing through a single AChR channel is 4 to 5 pA.[36,37] About 1000 to 2000 AChRs open in response to a quanta of ACh.[22,33] An EPC is about 200 nA, corresponding with about 50,000 AChR channels being open during an EPC.[22,33] The EPP for type IIb intercostal muscle fibers is about 40 mV.[29,30]

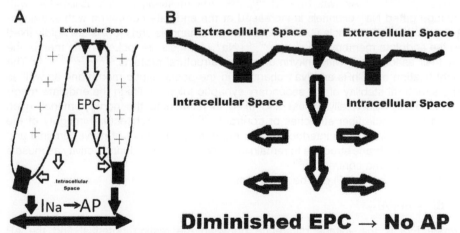

Fig. 2. Coupling of acetylcholine receptors (AChR) produced endplate current (EPC) and action potential (AP) generation. (*A*) At normal endplates the AChRs (▼) produce the EPC (*unfilled arrows*), which is directed by the secondary synaptic folds to the regions of high density of Na^+ channels (■) at the troughs of the synaptic folds exciting the Na^+ channels, which triggers an AP. (*B*) In myasthenia gravis the densities of AChR and Na^+ channels are reduced and secondary synaptic folds are diminished or absent. The EPC is smaller and the attenuated synaptic folds no longer guide the EPC to the Na^+ channels. The EPC is dissipated over a large membrane area. The dissipated EPC does not sufficiently activate Na+ channels to generate an AP.

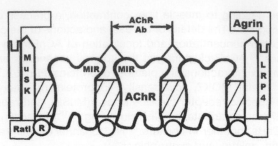

Fig. 3. Illustration of the acetylcholine receptor (AChR) clustering apparatus at the endplate. The structures include AChR, including the major immunogenic region, Agrin, the low-density lipoprotein receptor related protein 4, muscle-specific tyrosine kinase (MuSK), rapsyn and the rapsyn-associated linker protein (Ratl), which connects MuSK and rapsyn. The figure also shows how a divalent AChR antibody can cross-link 2 AChRs.

The concentration of AChRs at the endplate is about 1000-fold higher than the AChR concentration on extrajunctional membrane.[38] The relatively high concentration of AChRs at the endplate results because the muscle fiber nuclei near the endplate preferentially produce the messenger RNA encoding for AChR subunits.[39,40] AChRs continually turnover, with old receptors internalized and degraded. The removed receptors are replaced with new receptors. The AChRs are not recycled. Early in embryonic development, the half-life of AChRs is 13 to 24 hours.[41] At a mature endplate the half-life of AChRs is about 8 to 11 days. The cross-linking of receptors by antibodies dramatically shortens the AChR half-life by accelerating internalization of the receptors.[42,43]

Na^+ channels are concentrated in the depths of the secondary synaptic clefts.[22,27,35,44–51] As was true for AChRs, the messenger RNA associated with voltage-gated Na^+ channels is increased at the endplate compared with extrajunctional regions of a muscle fiber.[25] Both the Na^+ channels and AChRs are rigidly fixed in the endplate membrane.[30,35,39,40,46–53] Na^+ channels are locked in the membrane by their associations with ankyrin and other structural proteins.[24,27,31,35,40,47,52] The tight fixation of AChRs and Na^+ channels in the postsynaptic membrane as well as the structural stability of the secondary synaptic folds results in the endplate membrane being structurally robust and fixed in relation to the nerve terminal, even when the muscle fiber stretches or contracts.[30,53] The architectural integrity of the nerve terminal/endplate interface allows the critical alignment of nerve terminal and endplate membrane structure to remain in proper opposition during activity as muscle fibers stretch and contract.[30,53]

The safety factor (SF) can be defined as:

$$SF = EPP/E_{AP}$$

where E_{AP} is the voltage difference between the resting potential and the AP threshold.[54] The SF needs to be greater than 1 for an EPP to trigger an AP. The factors that contribute to the SF are (1) the amount of ACh released by the nerve terminal in response to an AP in the motor nerve fiber, (2) the sensitivity of the postsynaptic membrane to ACh, which is primarily dependent on the density of AChRs, (3) the high density of endplate Na^+ channels, which lowers the AP threshold at the endplate,[22,28–30,44,45,48–51,55,56] and (4) the presence of secondary synaptic folds, which greatly facilitate the coupling of the EPP to trigger APs.[22,26,30,31,33,57] The amount of ACh released combined with the high density of AChRs on the top of the secondary synaptic folds close to the release sites of ACh results in the EPP producing about a 40-mV depolarization in human intercostals muscle.[29,30] The high density of Na^+ channels at the endplate lowers the threshold for triggering an AP. The density of Na^+ channels at the endplate varies with fiber type.[48–51,55,56] Fast twitch fibers have about 500 to 550 Na^+ channels/μm^2 on the endplate membrane and slow twitch fibers have about 100 to 150 Na^+ channels/μm^2.[48–51]

The structure of the secondary synaptic folds greatly facilitates the electrical coupling between the EPP and AP. As shown in **Fig. 2**A, the depolarizing EPC associated with the EPP is directed by the secondary synaptic folds to the Na^+ channels at the base of the secondary synaptic folds.[22,29,30,32,33,57] If not for the secondary synaptic folds the EPC would enter the expansive muscle fiber cytosol and be dissipated over several millimeters of muscle length. The EPC would be too small to trigger an AP.[22,26,30,31,33,57] Wood and Slater[31] demonstrated that the synaptic folds in rat skeletal muscle double the SF. A physiologic measure of the dispersion of current or membrane potential is the space constant (λ). For current passing down a muscle fiber or junctional fold, the value of λ depends on the ratio of the transmembrane resistance to the internal resistance. The internal resistance or impedance measures how hard it is for current to pass through the cytosol. The transmembrane resistance or impedance is a measure of how hard it is for current to pass from the cytosol through the surface membrane to the extracellular space. The narrow diameter of a secondary synaptic fold results in a very high internal resistance. Current cannot easily pass through a lipid bilayer. Currents exit a cell by passing through ion pores or channels created by proteins. In the synaptic folds below the AChRs, the first available pathways for current to leave the cell are the Na^+ channels. The high internal resistance of secondary synaptic folds results in λ being small, only 0.435 μm. For human skeletal muscle, synaptic folds are about 1.5 μm long (Dr Andrew G. Engel, personal communication). The very small value for λ in a secondary synaptic fold indicates that 97% of the EPC current is dissipated within the synaptic fold. The Na^+ channels are the primary portals for current to exit the secondary synaptic folds. Therefore, almost all EPC goes to activating endplate Na^+ channels. If there were no secondary synaptic folds, the EPC would be dispersed through the 50 μm or greater diameter muscle fiber cytosol, with λ being about 1.5 μm.[53] The EPC dispersed over the surface membrane of a 1.5-μm length of muscle fiber would be too small to trigger an AP.[30]

EFFECTS OF ACETYLCHOLINE RECEPTORS ANTIBODIES IN MYASTHENIA GRAVIS

Early evidence that acquired myasthenia gravis (MG) was an autoimmune disease was the demonstration that serum immunoglobulins from people with MG bound to cytoplasmic cross-striational constituents of voluntary muscle cells.[58,59] Patrick and Lindstrom[60] made a major breakthrough in understanding the pathophysiology of MG when they observed that rabbits immunized with *Torpedo*-derived AChR developed weakness and neuromuscular electrophysiologic changes that resembled MG. Subsequent clinical studies demonstrated that antibodies directed against AChR cause MG.[61,62] About 80% to 85% of patients with MG have serum AChR antibodies that can be detected by radioimmunoprecipitation assay.[63–65] A greater fraction of patients with generalized MG have detectable AChR antibodies compared with those with ocular MG.

The endplate pathophysiology in MG is best understood for MG caused by AChR antibodies. The antibodies bind to AChRs and also damage endplate membrane. The nicotinic AChR at the innervated endplate is composed of 4 distinct membrane-spanning proteins or subunits referred to by Greek letters chosen by the chronologic order of subunit isolation, that is, α, β, δ, and ϵ.[37] Each AChR is composed of 5 subunits, 2 α-subunits and 1 copy of 3 other distinct subunits. Early in muscle fiber development and after denervation, muscle fiber express a fetal isoform of the AChR where the ϵ-subunit is replaced by a γ-subunit.[37] Each AChR has 2 binding sites for ACh. The α-subunit has a binding site for ACh, which extends into the junction region between the α-subunit and the δ-subunit for 1 binding site, and between the second α-subunit and the γ- or ϵ-subunit for the second binding site.[66] Pathogenic antibodies typically bind the extracellular regions of the AChR subunits. The α-subunit also contains a region called the main immunogenic region, which many antibodies target.[67,68] Antibodies reduce the effective number of endplate AChRs[42,61,69–72] by a combination of complement-mediated membrane lysis,[71] antibody binding to and interfering with AChR function, and acceleration of AChR breakdown and internalization resulting from antibodies cross-linking AChRs.[42,61,62,71,73]

MG can be induced in rats by immunization with foreign or self-AChR or by passive transfer of pathogenic AChR immunoglobulin (Ig)G (PTMG).[61,73–77] Weakness in PTMG begins about 12 hours after antibody injection and peaks at 48 hours.[75,76] After an initial period of prominent macrophage invasion, electrophysiologic and ultrastructural changes at the endplate are similar to those found in patients with autoimmune MG.[73,75,76]

ROLE OF COMPLEMENT IN ACETYLCHOLINE RECEPTORS MYASTHENIA GRAVIS

In the 1970s, Andrew Engel's laboratory demonstrated complement deposition at the endplate associated with AChR and endplate membrane loss in clinical MG and animal models of MG.[70,75,78–82] The importance of complement in endplate pathology was demonstrated by the dramatic effects of a component of cobra venom, which inhibits complement, to abrogate much of the endplate damage and many of the electrophysiologic changes in the passive transfer model of MG.[29,30,83] Complement inhibitors with greater clinical potential than cobra venom also reduced endplate damage in both passive transfer and active acquired experimental models of MG.[84–86] These experimental studies led to clinical trials with monoclonal antibodies directed against the C5 component of complement.[87,88]

Complement-mediated endplate damage in experiment and clinical MG results in the loss of endplate membrane, leading to a decrease in the length of the secondary synaptic folds, producing a simplified flattened postsynaptic membrane (**Fig. 2**B).[70,73,78,79,89] As discussed, synaptic folds contribute to the efficiency of coupling the EPP with triggering an AP. The importance of the loss of postsynaptic membrane in the pathophysiology of MG is supported by the observations that, although the serum level of AChR-binding antibodies do not predict the severity of weakness,[61,73,77] that postsynaptic membrane area correlates with the EPP size and with clinical signs of weakness.[70]

Complement-mediated endplate damage in experimental and clinical MG results in the loss of both AChRs and a lack of concentration of endplate Na^+ channels, which decreases the EPP and increases the threshold depolarization needed to trigger an AP.[28–30] The gating properties of Na^+ channels at the endplate and away from the endplate are not altered in MG or PTMG.[28–30] Additionally, the Na^+ current density away from the endplate is not changed in PTMG or MG.[28–30] Therefore, the pathogenic antibodies in MG and PTMG do not target Na^+ channels.[28–30] Na^+ channels are lost as "innocent bystanders," along with other membrane proteins owing to antibody-mediated membrane loss.[30] The decrease in EPP size and increase in AP threshold reduce the SF, with more severe MG being associated with a greater reduction in the SF.[30] The decrease in the EPP size and the increase in the AP threshold at the end-plate contribute about equally to the reduction in SF associated with MG.[30]

MYASTHENIA GRAVIS ASSOCIATED WITH ANTIBODIES TO MUSCLE-SPECIFIC RECEPTOR TYROSINE KINASE

About 15% of patients with generalized MG do not have serum detectable AChR antibodies by the standard radioimmunoprecipitation assay.[63,64,90] Serum from these "seronegative" patients can impair neuromuscular transmission in experimental settings.[90] Some of these seronegative patients have AChR antibodies that can be detected when tested using high-density clusters of AChRs.[63] However, the serum of other patients have antibodies that react to other components of the postsynaptic membrane. The first non-AChR antigenic target was MuSK.[91] MuSK antibodies are present in about 4% to 6% of people with MG.[64,65] Animal studies show that MuSK antibodies can cause muscle weakness by directly affecting the function of the neuromuscular junction[92,93]; therefore, MuSK antibodies are likely not simply disease markers in patients with MuSK MG.

The demographic and clinical features of AChR MG and MuSK MG usually differ. In the United States, MuSK MG is more common in African Americans compared with whites.[94] The clinical presentation of MuSK MG frequently, but not invariably, differs from AChR MG with regard to predominate distribution of weakness and severity.[95–98] In the rare double positive (AChR and MuSK positive) patients, the severity tends to be more like the MuSK patients, although admittedly the numbers of such patients are small.[99] MuSK MG has a stronger female predominance compared with AChR MG and is characterized by more frequent bulbar weakness and crises.[96,100] Additionally, in MuSK MG, patients are more likely to deteriorate rapidly early in the disease, plasma exchange seems more beneficial than intravenous antibody treatment, and patients with MuSK MG often do not respond to or are worsened by AChE inhibitor treatment.[96,100–103]

AChR antibodies are IgG classes 1 to 3, which are able to activate complement. In contrast, MuSK antibodies are predominantly of the IgG4 subclass, which does not fix complement.[104] The antigen-binding fragment (Fab) is the region of an antibody that binds to antigens. Each IgG antibody has 2 Fab chains. IgG4 antibodies are able to exchange Fab arms with other, unrelated, IgG4 antibodies. Therefore, IgG4 antibodies are potentially monovalent for a specific antigen.[105] In contrast, other IgG antibody classes are divalent, with both Fab segments directed to the same antigen. Divalent antibodies are able to cross-link targets such as the AChR (see **Fig. 3**), whereas monovalent antibodies cannot cross-link antigen targets. In AChR MG, the cross-linking of AChRs is associated with reduced AChR lifetimes.[42,43]

Given the important role of complement in AChR MG and the reduced capacity of MuSK antibodies to cross-link endplate proteins, how do MuSK antibodies cause disease? The pathologic mechanisms of MuSK antibodies are continuing to be elucidated, but several things are clear. First, one can create both active and passive transfer animal models of MuSK MG.[92,104,106–108] Second, both clinical and experimental MuSK MG shares several features associated with AChR MG, such as degeneration of the postsynaptic membrane with loss of AChRs and a reduction in the secondary synaptic fold length.[106] Both monovalent and divalent MuSK antibodies are pathogenic.[105,109] To our knowledge, complement does not cause endplate membrane damage in MuSK MG. Tüzün and colleagues[110] report increased complement breakdown in patients with MuSK MG, but the significance of this observation is not clear.

At present, MuSK antibodies are recognized to have 2 pathologic mechanisms. The first mechanism is that MuSK antibodies disrupt the normal interaction of essential proteins, including agrin, MuSK, LRP4, and rapsyn (see **Fig. 3**), which are involved in AChR membrane insertion, AChR clustering at the endplate, and the replacement of faulty AChRs.[104,107,108,111–114] LRP4 and MuSK function together on the postsynaptic membrane. Agrin binding to LRP4 triggers MuSK phosphorylation. Activated MuSK drives the clustering of AChRs.[16,115] When this postsynaptic protein network is disrupted, as occurs with MuSK antibodies,[104,107,108,111–114] the membrane does not properly insert and position AChRs and other membrane proteins. Mutations of MuSK causes congenital forms of MG characterized by disrupting AChR clustering and disruption other features of the complex organization of postsynaptic membrane.[113,116] To date, the density and properties of endplate Na^+ channels has not been studied in forms of acquired MG other than AChR MG.

The second action of MuSK MG antibodies is to disrupt the feedback between the nerve terminal and the endplate. In AChR MG or if one pharmacologically blocks AChRs, the nerve terminal attempts to compensate for the postsynaptic defect by increasing the quantal content, the number of vesicles of ACh released by the nerve terminal.[93,117] In MuSK MG, quantal content is not increased[93] and ACh release is compromised.[107,112,118,119] By mechanisms to be determined, the normal feedback between the nerve terminal and the endplate is disrupted in MuSK MG. Perhaps owing to the impaired release of ACh in MuSK MG, patients can benefit from 3,4-diaminopyridine, which increases quantal content by prolonging the duration of an AP in the nerve terminal so that more Ca^{2+} enters the nerve terminal leading to the release of more ACh vesicles.[120]

MuSK MG differs from AChR MG in that many patients with MuSK MG do not respond to or are worsened by pyridostigmine and other agents that inhibit AChE.[96,100–102,121] Electromyography reveals that patients develop repeated APs in response to AChE inhibitors,[102] which suggests that AChE inhibitor treatment in MuSK MG prolongs the duration of the EPP sufficiently to trigger multiple APs. One potential explanation for the abnormal AChE inhibitor response is that endplate Na^+ channels are not suppressed in MuSK MG. In AChR MG, the reduction in endplate Na^+ channels raises the AP threshold, which would prevent repeated APs forming in response to a prolonged EPP. The AChE molecule at the endplate has 2 components, a catalytic unit that hydrolyzes ACh and a long collagen tail. MuSK is one of the attachment sites for the collagen tail. Therefore, it is possible that the binding of MuSK antibodies inhibits the collagen tail from attaching to MuSK, leading to a deficiency of synaptic AChE. In a setting of reduced synaptic AChE, an AChE inhibitor could pathologically prolong the EPP leading to repeated APs in response to a single nerve impulse. The 2 suggested mechanisms are not mutually exclusive. A normal AP threshold at the endplate combined with a pathologically prolonged EPP could explain why AChE inhibitors trigger multiple APs in patients with MuSK MG. Multiple APs in response to a single nerve terminal impulse would disrupt normal motor function and could explain why many patients with MuSK MG do not tolerate AChE inhibitors.

LIPOPROTEIN RECEPTOR-RELATED PROTEIN 4 ANTIBODIES AND MYASTHENIA GRAVIS

Patients with clinical MG who do not have antibodies to AChR or MuSK (double seronegative) may have antibodies to LRP4.[122–125] Among double seronegative patients, the frequency of LRP4 antibodies varies greatly among different groups of people with a frequency of 18.7%[125] in one study and 4% in another.[126] Pathologic levels of antibodies to AChR and MuSK rarely, if ever, occur in the same patient, but antibodies to LRP4 were found in 8 of 107 patients with AChR MG and 10 of 67 patients with MuSK MG.[125] In contrast with MuSK MG, the antibodies of patients with LRP4 MG and in experimental LRP4 MG can fix complement.[122,125,127] However, LRP4 MG does not seem to have a strong complement-mediated pathogenic mechanism at the neuromuscular junction in either the experimental model or human MG. The reasons for this apparent disparity are not clear.

Data suggest that LRP4 antibodies are clinically significant rather than just markers of disease presence. First, LRP4 antibodies may be detected at MG symptom onset for patients, indicating that these antibodies were probably responsible for the muscle damage and not a reaction to muscle injury.[128] Immunization of C57BL/6 mice with LRP4 produced an MG-like condition with weakness and neuromuscular junction damage associated with LRP4 antibody and complement deposition on the endplate.[129] Experimental LRP4 MG antibodies were predominantly complement fixing IgG2 subclass. The importance of LRP4 in normal endplate development and maintenance is demonstrated in experimental settings where LRP4 is reduced, producing animals with weakness and neuromuscular damage that resembles MG.[93,130,131] LRP4 is expressed in nerve terminals and, as is true for MuSK, LRP4 contributes to feedback between the nerve terminal and the endplate membrane.[16,130,132] In a form of congenital MG associated with LRP4 mutations, the affected children had abnormally formed endplates, nerve terminal degeneration, and impaired neuromuscular transmission.[133]

OTHER POTENTIALLY PATHOGENIC ANTIBODIES

Antibodies against other endplate proteins have been identified in patients with clinical MG, but the clinicopathologic significance of the antibodies are not yet established. Zhang and colleagues[134] found antibodies to agrin in 7 serum samples from a group of patients with MG with known antibody status. Healthy controls and neurologic patients who did not have MG did not have agrin antibodies. Two of the 4 patients with MG who did not have antibodies to AChR, MuSK, or LRP4 had antibodies against agrin. Agrin antibodies were also found in 5 of 83 patients with AChR MG, but not in 6 patients with MuSK MG. None of the study group had LRP4 MG. Zhang and colleagues[134] reported that sera from the patients with agrin antibodies reacted with agrin and inhibited agrin-induced phosphorylation of MuSK and clustering of AChRs. These data suggest that agrin antibodies may be pathogenic, but further study is required.

Cortactin and Dok-7 are intracellular proteins involved with AChR clustering the assembly of the endplate membrane complex.[16,135] Cortés-Vicente and colleagues[65] studied 250 patients with MG from Spain. Cortactin antibodies were identified in 28 MG subjects: 9 of the 38 subjects who did not have AChR or MuSK antibodies and 19 of the 201 subjects who had AChR but not MuSK antibodies. None of the 11 subjects with MuSK MG or 29 controls had cortactin antibodies. However, an earlier report that included several of the same investigators found cortactin antibodies in 12.5% of patients with autoimmune diseases other than MG and 5.2% of healthy controls.[136] The pathologic potential of cortactin antibodies is unresolved at present. Antibodies against intracellular proteins involved with endplate assembly could be disease markers or modulators of disease severity rather than initiators of MG. Silencing Dok-7 in rats increases their susceptibility to passive transfer MG.[137] The roles of antibodies against the collagen tail of AChE antibodies in MG are being evaluated.[138] Antibodies to muscle intracellular proteins such as Titin may contribute to the severity of the disease but do not seem to be associated with impaired neuromuscular transmission.[139,140] As we are discovering in many autoimmune diseases, the autoantibody spectrum of each patient combined with immunoglobulin class of the antibodies appreciably influence clinical phenotype.[141,142]

SUMMARY

MG is associated with antibodies directed toward AChR, MuSK, and LRP4. In AChR MG, impaired neuromuscular transmission is associated with reduced EPP size and an increased threshold for generating an AP. Complement-mediated destruction of the endplate membrane is an important factor in AChR MG. MuSK MG does not seem to involve complement. Endplate damage seems to result from a disruption of the normal mechanisms for maintaining the endplate membrane. LRP4 MG may incorporate the pathogenic features associated with both AChR MG and MuSK MG because LRP4 antibodies can activate complement, and LRP4 is a critical element in the assembly and maintenance of the endplate membrane.

REFERENCES

1. Engel AG. The molecular biology of end-plate diseases. In: Salpeter MM, editor. The vertebrate neuromuscular junction, vol. 23. New York: Alan R. Liss, Inc; 1987. p. 361–424.

2. Smith SJ, Augustine GJ. Calcium ions, active zones and synaptic transmitter release. Trends Neurosci 1988;10:458–64.

3. Augustine GJ, Adler EM, Charlton MP. The calcium signal for transmitter secretion from presynaptic nerve terminals. Ann N Y Acad Sci 1991;635:365–81.

4. Protti DA, Sanchez VA, Cherksey BD, et al. Mammalian neuromuscular transmission blocked by funnel web toxin. Ann N Y Acad Sci 1993;681:405–7.

5. Miledi R, Molenaar PC, Polak RL. Electrophysiological and chemical determination of acetylcholine release at the frog neuromuscular junction. J Physiol 1983; 334:245–54.

6. Etcheberrigaray R, Fielder JL, Pollard HB, et al. Endoplasmic reticulum as a source of Ca^{2+} in neurotransmitter secretion. Ann N Y Acad Sci 1991;635:90–9.

7. Katz B, Miledi R. Estimates of quantal content during chemical potentiation of transmitter release. Proc R Soc Lond B Biol Sci 1979;205:369–78.

8. Land BR, Harris WV, Salpeter EE, et al. Diffusion and binding constants for acetylcholine derived from the falling phase of miniature endplate currents. Proc Natl Acad Sci U S A 1984;81:1594–8.

9. Katz B, Miledi R. The binding of acetylcholine to receptors and its removal from the synaptic cleft. J Physiol 1973;231:549–74.

10. McMahan UJ, Sanes JR, Marshall LM. Cholinesterase is associated with the basal lamina at the neuromuscular junction. Nature 1978;271:172–4.

11. Land BR, Salpeter EE, Salpeter MM. Kinetic parameters for acetylcholine interaction in intact neuromuscular junction. Proc Natl Acad Sci U S A 1981;78: 7200–4.

12. Colquhoun D, Sakmann B. Fast events in single-channel currents activated by acetylcholine and its analogues at the frog muscle end-plate. J Physiol 1985; 369:501–57.

13. Caputo C. Pharmacological investigations of excitation-contraction coupling. In: Peachy LD, Adrian RH, Geiger SR, editors. Handbook of physiology. Bethesda (MD): American Physiological Society; 1983. p. 381–415.

14. Donaldson SK. Mammalian muscle fiber types: comparison of excitation-contraction coupling mechanisms. Acta Physiol Scand 1986;128:157–66.

15. Beam KG, Horowicz P. Excitation-contraction coupling in skeletal muscle. In: Engel AG, Franzini-Armstrong C, editors. Myology, vol. 1, 3rd edition. New York: McGraw-Hill; 2004. p. 257–80.

16. Wu H, Xiong WC, Mei L. To build a synapse: signaling pathways in neuromuscular junction assembly. Development 2010;137:1017–33.

17. Luo Z, Wang Q, Dobbins GC, et al. Signaling complexes for postsynaptic differentiation. J Neurocytol 2003;32:697–708.

18. Gautam M, Noakes PG, Mudd J. Failure of postsynaptic specialization to at neuromuscular junctions of rapsyn-deficient mice. Nature 1995;377:232–6.

19. Gautam M, Noakes PG, Moscoso L. Defective neuromuscular synaptogenesis in agrin-deficient mutant mice. Cell 1996;85:525–35.

20. Holland PC, Carbonetto S. The extracellular matrix of skeletal muscle. In: Karpati G, Hilton-Jones D, Griggs RC, editors. Disorders of voluntary muscle. 7th edition. Cambridge (United Kingdom): Cambridge University Press; 2001. p. 103–21.

21. Vincent A. The neuromuscular junction and neuromuscular transmission. In: Karpati G, Hilton-Jones D, Griggs RC, editors. Disorders of voluntary muscle. 7th edition. Cambridge (United Kingdom): Cambridge University Press; 2001. p. 142–67.

22. Slater CR. Structural factors influencing the efficacy of neuromuscular transmission. Ann N Y Acad Sci 2008;1132:1–12.

23. Stocksley MA, Awad SS, Young C, et al. Accumulation of Nav1 mRNAs at differentiating postsynaptic sites in rat soleus muscles. Mol Cell Neurosci 2005;28(4): 694–702.

24. Bailey SJ, Stocksley MA, Buckel A, et al. Voltage-gated sodium channels and ankyrinG occupy a different postsynaptic domain from acetylcholine receptors from an early stage of neuromuscular junction maturation in rats. J Neurosci 2003;23(6):2102–11.

25. Awad SS, Lightowlers RN, Young C, et al. Sodium channel mRNAs at the neuromuscular junction: distinct patterns of accumulation and effects of muscle activity. J Neurosci 2001;21(21):8456–63.

26. Wood SJ, Slater CR. beta-Spectrin is colocalized with both voltage-gated sodium channels and ankyrinG at the adult rat neuromuscular junction. J Cell Biol 1998;140(3):675–84.

27. Caldwell JH. Clustering of sodium channels at the neuromuscular junction. Microsc Res Tech 2000;49(1):84–9.

28. Ruff RL, Lennon VA. Endplate voltage-gated sodium channels are lost in clinical and experimental myasthenia gravis. Ann Neurol 1998;43:370–9.

29. Ruff RL, Lennon VA. How myasthenia gravis alters the safety factor for neuromuscular transmission. J Neuroimmunol 2008;201-202:13–20.

30. Ruff RL. Endplate contributions to the safety factor for neuromuscular transmission. Muscle Nerve 2011;44:854–61.

31. Wood SJ, Slater CR. The contribution of postsynaptic folds to the safety factor for neuromuscular transmission in rat fast- and slow-twitch muscles. J Physiol 1997;500(1):165–76.

32. Slater CR, Lyons PR, Walls TJ, et al. Structure and function of neuromuscular junctions in the vastus lateralis of man. A motor point biopsy study of two groups of patients. Brain 1992;115:451–78.

33. Slater CR. Reliability of neuromuscular transmission and how it is maintained. Handb Clin Neurol 2008;91:27–101.

34. Slater CR, Fawcett PRW, Walls TJ, et al. Pre- and post-synaptic abnormalities associated with impaired neuromuscular transmission in a group of patients with 'limb-girdle myasthenia'. Brain 2006;129:2061–76.
35. Flucher BE, Daniels MP. Distribution of Na+ channels and ankyrin in neuromuscular junctions is complementary to that of acetylcholine receptors and the 43 kD protein. Neuron 1989;3:163–75.
36. Ruff RL. Ionic channels: I. The biophysical basis for ion passage and channel gating. Muscle Nerve 1986;9:675–99.
37. Ruff RL. Ionic channels II. Voltage- and agonist-gated and agonist-modified channel properties and structure. Muscle Nerve 1986;9:767–86.
38. Kuffler SW, Yoshikami D. The distribution of acetylcholine sensitivity at the post-synaptic membrane of vertebrate skeletal twitch muscles: iontophoretic mapping in the micron range. J Physiol 1975;244:703–30.
39. Merlie JP, Sanes JR. Concentration of acetylcholine receptor mRNA in synaptic regions of adult muscle fibers. Nature 1985;317:66–8.
40. Sanes JR, Johnson YR, Kotzbauer PT, et al. Selective expression of an acetylcholine receptor-lacZ transgene in synaptic nuclei of adult muscle fibers. Development 1991;113:1181–91.
41. Salpeter MM, Loring RH. Nicotinic acetylcholine receptors in vertebrate muscle: properties, distribution and neural control. Prog Neurobiol 1985;25:297–325.
42. Kao I, Drachman D. Myasthenic immunoglobulin accelerates acetylcholine receptor degradation. Science 1977;196:526–8.
43. Merlie JP, Heinemann S, Lindstrom JM. Acetylcholine receptor degradation in adult rat diaphragms in organ culture and the effect of anti-acetylcholine receptor antibodies. J Biol Chem 1979;254:6320–7.
44. Angelides KJ. Fluorescently labeled Na$^+$ channels are localized and immobilized to synapses of innervated muscle fibres. Nature 1986;321:63–6.
45. Le Teut T, Boudier J-L, Jover E, et al. Localization of voltage-sensitive sodium channels on the extrasynaptic membrane surface of mouse skeletal muscle by autoradiography of scorpion toxin binding sites. J Neurocytol 1990;19:408–20.
46. Haimovich B, Schotland DL, Fieles WE, et al. Localization of sodium channel subtypes in rat skeletal muscle using channel-specific monoclonal antibodies. J Neurosci 1987;7:2957–66.
47. Roberts WM. Sodium channels near end-plates and nuclei of snake skeletal muscle. J Physiol 1987;388:213–32.
48. Ruff RL. Na current density at and away from end plates on rat fast- and slow-twitch skeletal muscle fibers. Am J Physiol 1992;262(1 Pt 1):C229–34.
49. Ruff RL, Whittlesey D. Na$^+$ current densities and voltage dependence in human intercostal muscle fibres. J Physiol 1992;458:85–97.
50. Ruff RL, Whittlesey D. Na$^+$ currents near and away from endplates on human fast and slow twitch muscle fibers. Muscle Nerve 1993;16:922–9.
51. Ruff RL, Whittlesey D. Comparison of Na$^+$ currents from type IIa and IIb human intercostal muscle fibers. Am J Physiol 1993;265(1 Pt 1):C171–7.
52. Martinou JC, Falls DI, Fischback GD, et al. Acetylcholine receptor-inducing activity stimulates expression of the epsilon-subunit gene of the muscle acetylcholine receptor. Proc Natl Acad Sci U S A 1991;88:7669–73.
53. Ruff RL. Effects of length changes on Na$^+$ current amplitude and excitability near and far from the end-plate. Muscle Nerve 1996;19:1084–92.
54. Katz B. Nerve muscle and synapse. New York: McGraw-Hill Co; 1966.
55. Caldwell JH, Campbell DT, Beam KG. Sodium channel distribution in vertebrate skeletal muscle. J Gen Physiol 1986;87:907–32.

56. Milton RL, Lupa MT, Caldwell JH. Fast and slow twitch skeletal muscle fibres differ in their distributions of Na channels near the endplate. Neurosci Lett 1992;135:41–4.
57. Wood SJ, Slater CR. Safety factor at the neuromuscular junction. Prog Neurobiol 2001;64(4):393–429.
58. Strauss AJ, Smith CW, Cage GW, et al. Further studies on the specificity of presumed immune associations of myasthenia gravis and consideration of possible pathogenic implications. Ann N Y Acad Sci 1966;135:557–79.
59. Strauss AJ, van der Geld HW, Kemp PG, et al. Immunological concomitants of myasthenia gravis. Ann N Y Acad Sci 1965;124:744–66.
60. Patrick J, Lindstrom J. Autoimmune response to acetylcholine receptor. Science 1973;180:871–2.
61. Drachman DB. Myasthenia gravis. N Engl J Med 1994;330:1797–810.
62. Vincent A, McConville J, Farrugia MA, et al. Autoantibodies in myasthenia gravis and related disorders. Ann N Y Acad Sci 2003;998:324–35.
63. Leite MI, Jacob S, Viegas S, et al. IgG1 antibodies to acetylcholine receptors in 'seronegative' myasthenia gravis. Brain 2008;131(Pt 7):1940–52.
64. Chang T, Leite MI, Senanayake S, et al. Clinical and serological study of myasthenia gravis using both radioimmunoprecipitation and cell-based assays in a South Asian population. J Neurol Sci 2014;342(1–2):82–7.
65. Cortés-Vicente E, Gallardo E, Martínez MÁ, et al. Clinical characteristics of patients with double-seronegative myasthenia gravis and antibodies to cortactin. JAMA Neurol 2016;73(9):1099–104.
66. Unwin N. Projection structure of the nicotinic acetylcholine receptor: distinct conformations of the α subunits. J Mol Biol 1996;257:586–96.
67. Lennon VA, McCormick DJ, Lambert E, et al. Region of peptide 125-147 of acetylcholine receptor alpha subunit is exposed at neuromuscular junction and induces experimental autoimmune myasthenia gravis, T-cell immunity, and modulating autoantibodies. Proc Natl Acad Sci U S A 1985;82:8805–9.
68. Fostieri E, Beeson D, Tzartos SJ. The conformation of the main immunogenic region on the alpha-subunit of muscle acetylcholine receptor is affected by neighboring receptor subunits. FEBS Lett 2000;481(2):127–30.
69. Fambrough DM, Drachman DB, Satyamurti S. Neuromuscular junction in myasthenia gravis: decreased acetylcholine receptors. Science 1973;182:293–5.
70. Engel AG, Lindstrom JM, Lambert EH, et al. Ultrastructural localization of the acetylcholine receptors in myasthenia gravis and in its experimental autoimmune model. Neurology 1977;27:307–15.
71. Engel AG, Fumagalli G. Mechanisms of acetylcholine receptor loss from the neuromuscular junction. Ciba Found Symp 1982;90:197–224.
72. Kaminski HJ, Ruff RL. Structure and kinetic properties of the acetylcholine receptor. In: Engel AG, editor. Myasthenia gravis and myasthenic syndromes, vol. 56. New York: Oxford University Press; 1999. p. 40–64.
73. Engel AG. Acquired autoimmune myasthenia gravis. In: Engel AG, Franzini-Armstrong C, editors. Myology. 2nd edition. New York: McGraw-Hill; 1994. p. 1769–97.
74. Lindstrom JM, Einarson BL, Lennon VA, et al. Pathological mechanisms in experimental autoimmune myasthenia gravis. I. Immunogenicity of syngeneic muscle acetylcholine receptor and quantitative extraction of receptor and anti-receptor complexes from muscle of rats with experimental autoimmune myasthenia gravis. J Exp Med 1976;144:726–38.

75. Lindstrom JM, Engel AG, Seybold ME, et al. Pathological mechanisms in experimental autoimmune myasthenia gravis. II. Passive transfer of experimental autoimmune myasthenia gravis in rats with anti-acetylcholine receptor antibodies. J Exp Med 1976;144:739–53.
76. Lennon VA, Lambert EH. Myasthenia gravis induced by monoclonal antibodies to acetylcholine receptors. Nature 1980;285:238–40.
77. Kaminski HJ, Ruff RL. The myasthenic syndromes. In: Schultz SG, Andreoli TE, Brown AM, et al, editors. Physiology of membrane disorders, vol. 1, 2nd edition. New York: Plenum Press; 1996. p. 565–93.
78. Engel AG, Santa T. Histometric analysis of the ultrastructure of the neuromuscular junction in myasthenia gravis and the myasthenic syndrome. Ann N Y Acad Sci 1971;183:46–63.
79. Santa T, Engel AG, Lambert EH. Histometric study of neuromuscular junction ultrastructure. I. Myasthenia gravis. Neurology 1972;22:71–82.
80. Engel AG, Tsujihata M, Lindstrom JM, et al. The motor end plate in myasthenia gravis and in experimental autoimmune myasthenia gravis. A quantitative ultrastructural study. Ann N Y Acad Sci 1976;274:60–79.
81. Engel AG, Lambert EH, Howard FM. Immune complexes (IgG and C3) at the motor end-plate in myasthenia gravis. Ultrastructure and light microscopic localization and electrophysiological correlations. Mayo Clin Proc 1977;52:267–80.
82. Engel AG, Sakakibara H, Sahashi K, et al. Passively transferred experimental autoimmune myasthenia gravis. Sequential and quantitative study of the motor end-plate fine structure and ultrastructural localization of immune complexes (IgG and C3), and of the acetylcholine receptor. Neurology 1979;29:179–88.
83. Lennon VA, Seybold ME, Lindstrom JM, et al. Role of complement in the pathogenesis of experimental autoimmune myasthenia gravis. J Exp Med 1978;147:973–83.
84. Zhou Y, Gong B, Lin F, et al. Anti-C5 antibody treatment ameliorates weakness in experimentally acquired myasthenia gravis. J Immunol 2007;179(12):8562–7.
85. Soltys J, Kusner LL, Young A, et al. Novel complement inhibitor limits severity of experimentally induced myasthenia gravis. Ann Neurol 2009;65(1):67–75.
86. Kusner LL, Satija N, Cheng G, et al. Targeting therapy to the neuromuscular junction: proof of concept. Muscle Nerve 2014;49(5):749–56.
87. Howard JF, Freimer M, O'brien F, et al. QMG and MG-ADL correlations: study of eculizumab treatment of myasthenia gravis. Muscle Nerve 2017;56(2):328–30.
88. Howard JF, Utsugisawa K, Benatar M, et al. Safety and efficacy of eculizumab in anti-acetylcholine receptor antibody-positive refractory generalized myasthenia gravis (REGAIN): a phse 3, randomized, double-blind, placebo-controlled, multicentre study. Lancet Neurol 2017;16:886–976.
89. Maselli RA, Richman DP, Wollmann RL. Inflammation at the neuromuscular junction in myasthenia gravis. Neurology 1991;41:1497–504.
90. Mossman S, Vincent A, Newsom-Davis J. Myasthenia gravis without acetylcholine receptor antibody: a distinct disease entity. Lancet 1986;1(8473):116–9.
91. Hoch W, McConville J, Helms S, et al. Auto-antibodies to the receptor tyrosine kinase MuSK in patients with myasthenia gravis without acetylcholine receptor antibodies. Nat Med 2001;7(3):365–8.
92. Phillips WD, Christadoss P, Losen M, et al. Guidelines for pre-clinical animal and cellular models of MuSK-myasthenia gravis. Exp Neurol 2015;270:29–40.
93. Plomp JJ, Morsch M, Phillips WD, et al. Electrophysiological analysis of neuromuscular synaptic function in myasthenia gravis patients and animal models. Exp Neurol 2015;270:41–54.

94. Oh SJ, Morgan MB, Lu L, et al. Different characteristic phenotypes according to antibody in myasthenia gravis. J Clin Neuromuscul Dis 2012;14(2):57–65.
95. Evoli A, Tonali PA, Padua L, et al. Clinical correlates with anti-MuSK antibodies in generalized seronegative myasthenia gravis. Brain 2003;126:2304–11.
96. Guptill JT, Sanders DB, Evoli A. Anti-MuSK antibody myasthenia gravis: clinical findings and response to treatment in two large cohorts. Muscle Nerve 2011; 44(1):36–40.
97. McConville J, Farrugia ME, Beeson D, et al. Detection and characterization of MuSK antibodies in seronegative myasthenia gravis. Ann Neurol 2004;55: 580–4.
98. Sanders DB, El-Salem K, Massey JM, et al. Clinical aspects of MuSK antibody positive seronegative MG. Neurology 2003;60:1978–80.
99. Hong Y, Zisimopoulou P, Trakas N, et al. Multiple antibody detection in 'seroneg-ative' myasthenia gravis patients. Eur J Neurol 2017;24:844–50.
100. Pasnoor M, Wolfe GI, Nations S, et al. Clinical findings in MuSK-antibody positive myasthenia gravis: a U.S. experience. Muscle Nerve 2010;41(3):370–4.
101. El-Salem K, Yassin A, Al-Hayk K, et al. Treatment of MuSK-associated myasthenia gravis. Curr Treat Options Neurol 2014;16(4):283–8.
102. Shin HY, Park HJ, Lee HE, et al. Clinical and electrophysiologic responses to acetylcholinesterase inhibitors in MuSK-antibody-positive myasthenia gravis: evidence for cholinergic neuromuscular hyperactivity. J Clin Neurol 2014; 10(2):119–24.
103. Melzer N, Ruck T, Fuhr P, et al. Clinical features, pathogenesis, and treatment of myasthenia gravis: a supplement to the Guidelines of the German Neurological Society. J Neurol 2016;263(8):1473–94.
104. Plomp JJ, Huijbers MG, van der Maarel SM, et al. Pathogenic IgG4 subclass autoantibodies in MuSK myasthenia gravis. Ann N Y Acad Sci 2012;1275:114–22.
105. Koneczny I, Stevens JA, De Rosa A, et al. IgG4 autoantibodies against muscle-specific kinase undergo Fab-arm exchange in myasthenia gravis patients. J Autoimmun 2017;77:104–15.
106. Richman DP, Nishi K, Morell SW, et al. Acute severe animal model of anti–muscle-specific kinase myasthenia combined postsynaptic and presynaptic changes. Arch Neurol 2012;69(4):453–60.
107. Viegas S, Jacobson L, Waters P, et al. Passive and active immunization models of MuSK-Ab positive myasthenia: electrophysiological evidence for pre and postsynaptic defects. Exp Neurol 2012;234(2):506–12.
108. Huijbers MG, Zhang W, Klooster R, et al. MuSK IgG4 autoantibodies cause myasthenia gravis by inhibiting binding between MuSK and Lrp4. Proc Natl Acad Sci U S A 2013;110(51):20783–8.
109. Mori S, Yamada S, Kubo S, et al. Divalent and monovalent autoantibodies cause dysfunction of MuSK by distinct mechanisms in a rabbit model of myasthenia gravis. J Neuroimmunol 2012;244(1–2):1–7.
110. Tüzün E, Yilmaz V, Parman Y, et al. Increased complement consumption in MuSK-antibody-positive myasthenia gravis patients. Med Princ Pract 2011;20: 581–3.
111. Punga AR, Lin S, Oliveri F, et al. Muscle-selective synaptic disassembly and reorganization in MuSK antibody positive MG mice. Exp Neurol 2011;230(2): 207–17.
112. Mori S, Kubo S, Akiyoshi T, et al. Antibodies against muscle-specific kinase impair both presynaptic and postsynaptic functions in a murine model of myasthenia gravis. Am J Pathol 2012;180(2):798–810.

113. Otsuka K, Ito M, Ohkawara B, et al. Collagen Q and anti-MuSK autoantibody competitively suppress agrin/LRP4/MuSK signaling. Sci Rep 2015;10(5):13928.
114. Ohno K, Otsuka K, Ito M. Roles of collagen Q in MuSK antibody-positive myasthenia gravis. Chem Biol Interact 2016;259(Pt. B):266–70.
115. Mazhar S, Herbst R. The formation of complex acetylcholine receptor clusters requires MuSK kinase activity and structural information from the MuSK extracellular domain. Mol Cell Neurosci 2012;49(4):475–86.
116. Gallenmüller C, Müller-Felber W, Dusl M, et al. Salbutamol-responsive limb-girdle congenital myasthenic syndrome due to a novel missense mutation and heteroallelic deletion in MuSK. Neuromuscul Disord 2014;24:31–5.
117. Plomp JJ, Van Kempen GT, De Baets MB, et al. Acetylcholine release in myasthenia gravis: regulation at single end-plate level. Ann Neurol 1995;37(5):627–36.
118. Chroni E, Punga AR. Neurophysiological characteristics of MuSK antibody positive myasthenia gravis mice: focal denervation and hypersensitivity to acetylcholinesterase inhibitors. J Neurol Sci 2012;316(1–2):150–7.
119. Patel V, Oh A, Voit A, et al. Altered active zones, vesicle pools, nerve terminal conductivity, and morphology during experimental MuSK myasthenia gravis. PLoS One 2014;9(12):e110571.
120. Mori S, Kishi M, Kubo S, et al. 3,4-Diaminopyridine improves neuromuscular transmission in a MuSK antibody-induced mouse model of myasthenia gravis. J Neuroimmunol 2012;245(1–2):75–80.
121. Morsch M, Reddel SW, Ghazanfari N, et al. Pyridostigmine but not 3,4-diaminopyridine exacerbates ACh receptor loss and myasthenia induced in mice by muscle-specific kinase autoantibody. J Physiol 2013;591(10):2747–62.
122. Higuchi O, Hamuro J, Motomura M, et al. Autoantibodies to low-density lipoprotein receptor-related protein 4 in myasthenia gravis. Ann Neurol 2011;69(2):418–22.
123. Pevzner A, Schoser B, Peters K, et al. Anti-LRP4 autoantibodies in AChR- and MuSK-antibody-negative myasthenia gravis. J Neurol Sci 2012;259(3):427–35.
124. Zhang B, Tzartos JS, Belimezi M, et al. Autoantibodies to lipoprotein-related protein 4 in patients with double-seronegative myasthenia gravis. Arch Neurol 2012;69(4):445–51.
125. Zisimopoulou P, Evangelakou P, Tzartos J, et al. A comprehensive analysis of the epidemiology and clinical characteristics of anti-LRP4 in myasthenia gravis. J Autoimmun 2014;52:139–45.
126. Li Y, Zhang Y, Cai G, et al. Anti-LRP4 autoantibodies in Chinese patients with myasthenia gravis. Muscle Nerve 2017;56(5):938–42.
127. Shen C, Lu Y, Zhang B, et al. Antibodies against low-density lipoprotein receptor-related protein 4 induce myasthenia gravis. J Clin Invest 2013;123:5190–202.
128. Zouvelou V, Zisimopoulou P, Rentzos M, et al. Double seronegative myasthenia gravis with anti-LRP 4 antibodies. Neuromuscul Disord 2013;23(7):568–70.
129. Ulusoy C, Çavus F, Yilmaz V, et al. Immunization with recombinantly expressed LRP4 induces experimental autoimmune myasthenia gravis in C57BL/6 mice. Immunol Invest 2017;4:1–10.
130. Wu H, Lu Y, Shen C, et al. Distinct roles of muscle and motoneuron LRP4 in neuromuscular junction formation. Neuron 2012;75(1):94–107.
131. Takamori M. Synaptic homeostasis and its immunological disturbance in neuromuscular junction disorders. Int J Mol Sci 2017;18(4) [pii:E896].

132. Yumoto N, Kim N, Burden SJ. Lrp4 is a retrograde signal for presynaptic differentiation at neuromuscular synapses. Nature 2012;489:438–42.
133. Selcen D, Ohkawara B, Shen XM, et al. Impaired synaptic development, maintenance, and neuromuscular transmission in LRP4-related myasthenia. JAMA Neurol 2015;72(8):889–96.
134. Zhang B, Shen C, Bealmear B, et al. Autoantibodies to agrin in myasthenia gravis patients. PLoS One 2014;9(3):e91816.
135. Proszynski TJ, Gingras J, Valdez G, et al. Podosomes are present in a postsynaptic apparatus and participate in its maturation. Proc Natl Acad Sci U S A 2009;106(43):18373–8.
136. Gallardo E, Martínez-Hernández E, Titulaer MJ, et al. Cortactin autoantibodies in myasthenia gravis. Autoimmun Rev 2014;13(10):1003–7.
137. Gomez AM, Stevens JA, Mané-Damas M, et al. Silencing of Dok-7 in adult rat muscle increases susceptibility to passive transfer myasthenia gravis. Am J Pathol 2016;186(10):2559–68.
138. Zoltowska Katarzyna M, Belaya K, Leite M, et al. Collagen Q–a potential target for autoantibodies in myasthenia gravis. J Neurol Sci 2015;348:241–4.
139. Romi F, Skeie GO, Aarli JA, et al. The severity of myasthenia gravis correlates with the serum concentration of titin and ryanodine receptor antibodies. Arch Neurol 2000;57:1596–600.
140. Romi F, Skeie GO, Vedeler C, et al. Complement activation by titin and ryanodine receptor autoantibodies in myasthenia gravis. A study of IgG subclasses and clinical correlations. J Neuroimmunol 2000;111:169–76.
141. Meriggioli MN, Sanders DB. Autoimmune myasthenia gravis: emerging clinical and biological heterogeneity. Lancet Neurol 2009;8:475–90.
142. Meriggioli MN, Sanders DB. Muscle autoantibodies in myasthenia gravis: beyond diagnosis? Expert Rev Clin Immunol 2012;8:427–38.

Muscle-Specific Tyrosine Kinase and Myasthenia Gravis Owing to Other Antibodies

Michael H. Rivner, MD[a],*, Mamatha Pasnoor, MD[b],
Mazen M. Dimachkie, MD[c], Richard J. Barohn, MD[d], Lin Mei, PhD[e]

KEYWORDS

• Myasthenia gravis • MuSK • Cortactin • Agrin • LRP4 • Rapsyn

KEY POINTS

• Approximately 20% of patients with myasthenia gravis are acetylcholine receptor negative; in some, antibodies to proteins responsible for the maintenance of the neuromuscular junction have been found.

• Muscle-specific tyrosine kinase antibodies are found in around 30% to 40% of patients with double-negative myasthenia gravis.

• Muscle-specific tyrosine kinase positive patients generally respond well to immunosuppressive therapy and rituximab, but may not respond to pyridostigmine.

• Low-density lipoprotein receptor-related protein 4 antibodies are present in around 18% of patients with double-negative myasthenia gravis, and there is evidence that these antibodies are pathogenic.

• The role of antibodies to agrin, rapsyn, and cortactin in myasthenia gravis are not well-defined at present and further research is needed.

INTRODUCTION

Acetylcholine receptor (AChR) antibodies are found in approximately 80% of patients with myasthenia gravis (MG), leaving approximately 20% with antibody negative MG (SNMG).[1] It was suspected that patients with SNMG had an autoimmune etiology because they responded to autoimmune therapy, including plasma exchange.[2,3] In

---

Disclosure Statement: See last page of article.
[a] EMG Lab, Augusta University, 1120 15th Street, BP-4390, Augusta, GA 30912, USA;
[b] Department of Neurology, University of Kansas Medical Center, 3901 Rainbow Boulevard, Kansas City, KS 66160, USA; [c] Department of Neurology, University of Kansas Medical Center, 3599 Rainbow Boulevard, Mail Stop 2012, Kansas City, KS 66103, USA; [d] Department of Neurology, University of Kansas Medical Center, 3901 Rainbow Boulevard, Mail Stop 4017, Kansas City, KS 66160, USA; [e] Department of Neuroscience and Regenerative Medicine, Augusta University, 1120 15th Street, CA-2014, Augusta, GA 30912, USA
* Corresponding author.
E-mail address: MRIVNER@augusta.edu

Neurol Clin 36 (2018) 293–310
https://doi.org/10.1016/j.ncl.2018.01.004
0733-8619/18/© 2018 Elsevier Inc. All rights reserved.

addition, the passive transfer of disease to mice from the serum of seronegative patients,[2,4] the development of transient neonatal myasthenia in infants of seronegative myasthenic women,[5–7] and the binding of immunoglobulin (Ig)G from patients with seronegative MG to muscle[8] suggest an autoimmune etiology. In 2001, Hoch and colleagues[9] discovered that antibodies to muscle-specific tyrosine kinase (MuSK) were responsible for producing MG in about 70% of these patients with SNMG. More recently antibodies to low-density lipoprotein receptor-related protein 4 (LRP4)[10–12] and agrin[13,14] have been discovered in patients with MG. Other antibodies including titin,[15,16] cortactin,[17] and rapsyn[18] are associated with MG. Defects of these proteins are associated with congenital myasthenic syndromes.[19–34] The functions of these newly identified target proteins differ from AChR because they are responsible for the proper formation and maintenance of the neuromuscular junction rather than serving as AChR. In this article, we discuss the roles of these proteins and the known features of myasthenic patients who have antibodies to them.

When muscles are denervated, there is a significant alteration at the neuromuscular junction, including the expression of fetal AChR remote from the neuromuscular junction and increased muscle sensitivity to acetylcholine. With reinnervation, neuromuscular junctions are reformed, and the fetal AChR are eliminated as normal sensitivity to acetylcholine returns. This finding indicates that muscles are innervated and receive signals from motor neuron terminals. In addition, denervated muscle attracts neighboring neurons to sprout and form new connections. Agrin, a heparin sulfate proteoglycan[35] that is released by the axon terminal, plays an important role in the development and maintenance of neuromuscular junctions. The activation of MuSK, anchored in skeletal muscle, is responsible for the clustering of AChR at the neuromuscular junction. Although it is known that agrin is necessary for the activation of MuSK, there is no direct interaction between agrin and MuSK. In the last decade, LRP4[36,37] was discovered to be the agrin receptor that is responsible for activating MuSK. Agrin signaling, including MuSK and LRP4, have additional roles in inhibiting neurite outgrowth,[38] which may be responsible for the inhibition of sprouting. In addition, MuSK along with ColQ is responsible for anchoring acetylcholinesterase to the neuromuscular junction.[39–41]

Fig. 1 illustrates that interaction between the axon terminal and muscle. Agrin released by the axon terminal binds to LRP4 in muscles to activate MuSK. The formation of an agrin-LRP4 tetrameric complex (2 agrin molecules and 2 LRP4 molecules) is critical for MuSK activation.[42] DOK7, a muscle cytoplasmic protein, is also involved in

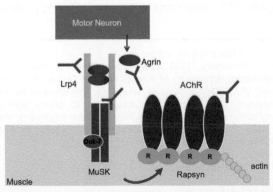

Fig. 1. Structure of the neuromuscular junction. AChR, acetylcholine receptor; Lrp4, low-density lipoprotein receptor-related protein 4; MuSK, muscle-specific tyrosine kinase.

the activation of MuSK.[43–46] Activated MuSK interacts with rapsyn, a scaffolding protein,[47–52] causing the clustering of AChR at the neuromuscular junction. Rapsyn binds all subunits of the AChR[51,53] and is bound to actin.[54] For a further review of the molecular anatomy of the neuromuscular junction as we well as the electrophysiological properties, the reader is referred to Robert L. Ruff and Robert P. Lisak's article, "Nature and Action of Antibodies in Myasthenia Gravis," in this issue. These elements of the neuromuscular junction are necessary for its proper development and maintenance. In addition to these actions, LRP4, agrin and MuSK act on the axonal terminal. Congenital defects of these proteins are linked to defects in neuromuscular transmission, and are discussed further in Perry B. Shieh and Shin J. Oh's article, "Congenital Myasthenia Syndromes," in this issue. Although there are many proteins of the neuromuscular junction that might be susceptible to antibodies, it is those that are exposed to the extracellular space namely agrin, LRP4, MuSK, and AChR, that are most likely to be vulnerable.

MUSCLE-SPECIFIC TYROSINE KINASE ANTIBODY-POSITIVE MYASTHENIA GRAVIS

MuSK was first described by Valenzuela and colleagues[55] in 1995 and was localized to the postjunction region of the neuromuscular junction. MuSK was shown to be involved in agrin signaling, causing the aggregation of AChRs at the neuromuscular junction.[56,57] In 2001, Hoch and colleagues[9] described 17 cases of MuSK antibody-positive MG out of 24 patients with SNMG. IgG from MuSK antibody-positive patients produce MG-like symptoms, including muscle weakness and destruction of the neuromuscular junction, when injected into mice.[58] Mice who developed anti-MuSK antibodies after being injected with rat MuSK acquire symptoms consistent with MG, including weakness, a decrement to repetitive stimulation, and reduced amplitude miniature endplate potentials.[59] MuSK antibodies produce wasting of muscles when injected in mice with a predilection to the masseter and facial muscles,[60] which might explain why these muscles are more involved clinically. Around 7% to 10% of all patients with MG have antibodies to MuSK. Initially, Hoch and colleagues[9] reported MuSK antibodies in 70% of AChR antibody–negative cases. However, subsequently most believe that this figure is closer to 30% to 40%.[61,62] Early studies indicate that patients with MuSK antibody-positive MG have important clinical differences when compared with AChR antibody-positive MG.[63,64] These patients have more bulbar, neck, and respiratory symptoms along with fewer ocular symptoms. The patients are less responsive to cholinesterase inhibitors, but responded to plasma exchange and other immunosuppressant medications.

Based on 16 years of experience, clinicians now recognize some characteristic features of MuSK antibody-positive MG. They are more likely to be female than male[65]; blacks are more likely to have these antibodies compared with whites.[66–68] There is considerable variation of the incidence of MuSK antibody-positive MG depending on geographic location.[66,69–71] Anti-MuSK antibody positive patients have HLA-DRB1, -DQB1, -DQ5, and -DR14 alleles.[72–74] Patients have marked bulbar weakness,[65] often with marked wasting and fasciculations of the tongue, and must be distinguished from patients with bulbar amyotrophic lateral sclerosis.[75,76] They often have facial, neck, and respiratory weakness. Their ocular symptoms are less prominent than other patients with MG. They are less likely to respond to anticholinesterase medication, perhaps because of deficient binding of acetylcholinesterase to the neuromuscular junction.[77,78] In addition to a case report,[79] our experience suggests that, although only 16% of patients with MuSK MG respond to cholinesterase inhibitors, hypersensitivity or worsening of symptoms occurred in 20% of cases.[76]

Others have also reported worsening symptoms in response to cholinesterase inhibitors in 5% of MuSK MG cases, whereas 57% improved.[80]

A patient of one of the authors (M.H.R.) illustrates a typical case of MuSK antibody positive MG. He is a 50-year-old black man who was in his usual state until he developed a flulike illness. He displayed dysarthria, swelling of the tongue, facial weakness, and bilateral ptosis, but without diplopia. He lost 50 pounds over a 3-month period. He noticed some weakness of his right shoulders, which became worse later in the day. A computed tomography scan of the chest scan was normal. Pulmonary function tests showed mild restrictive airway disease. Pyridostigmine produced little improvement of his symptoms; however, prednisone improved his symptoms. On examination, the patient had moderate ptosis without fatigue, with 4 out of 5 strength of his orbicularis oculi and 4+ out of 5 for the strength of the orbicularis oris (**Fig. 2**A). He was unable to wrinkle his brow (**Fig. 2**B), his voice was dysarthric, and there was mild weakness of his uvula. His tongue exhibited moderate wasting, fasciculations, and had mildly slowed rapid alternating movements (**Fig. 2**C). His neck and limbs were normal as was the remainder of his examination. He was Myasthenia Gravis Foundation of America (MGFA) Class[81] IIIb at his worst. He was negative for AChR and antistriatal muscle antibodies, but anti-MuSK antibodies were markedly elevated at 5.91 (normal, <0.03). Repetitive stimulation of his left facial nerve was normal, but needle examination revealed a slightly increased insertional activity of his orbicularis oculi with markedly diminished motor unit size with short duration motor units. Other muscles studied were normal. Stimulated single fiber electromyography of the right orbicularis oculi was very abnormal, with an average MCD of 260 μs with 80% of the fibers having blocks.

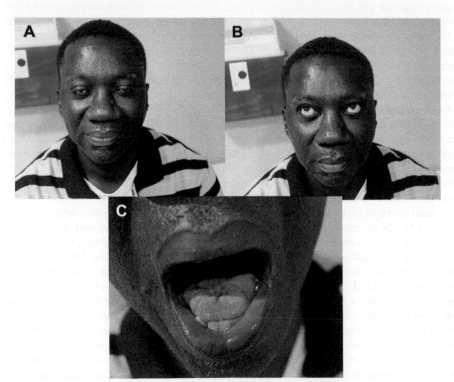

Fig. 2. Patient with anti–muscle-specific tyrosine kinase myasthenia gravis. (*A*) showing bilateral ptosis at rest. (*B*) unable to wrinkle brow on upward gaze. (*C*) tongue wasting.

Although patients with MuSK antibody-positive MG have less prominent ocular findings compared with AChR antibody-positive MG, cases of patients with pure ocular and predominantly ocular disease are described.[82–87] Cases of isolated neck weakness and wasting are described associated with anti-MuSK antibodies.[63,88–90] In addition, mutations of the MuSK protein have been associated with dropped head.[91] Vocal cord paralysis is seen in some patients with MuSK antibody-positive MG.[92–94] Although most patients just have anti-MuSK antibodies, patients with antibodies to MuSK and AChR[95,96] and voltage-gated calcium channels[97,98] are described. The anti-MuSK antibody level is generally correlated with symptoms.[99] MuSK antibodies have crossed the placenta in pregnant women, producing neonatal myasthenia.[100–104] Guptill and Sanders[105] described 3 different clinical presentations of MuSK antibody-positive MG. First, patients with predominantly bulbar and respiratory symptoms; second, patients indistinguishable from AChR antibody-positive MG; and third, patients presenting with head drop as their most prominent symptom. The above described MuSK antibody-positive MG patient was an example of the first clinical presentation pattern. Although thymic pathology including thymoma has been described in patients with MuSK antibody-positive MG,[106–108] this finding is far less common than in AChR antibody-positive MG.[64,67,109–111] It is unknown if thymectomy is of any value in these patients.[63,78] In the case series reported by Pasnoor and colleagues,[76] some patients with MuSK MG who had thymectomy did improve over time. Because several other therapies were also being administered, we cannot definitively say that thymectomy was the driver behind their improvement.[76] There have been reports of patients who initially presented as AChR antibody positive and, after thymectomies, developed MuSK antibody-positive MG.[96,112–115]

Patients with MuSK antibody-positive MG are more likely to have abnormal repetitive nerve studies in facial and proximal limb than in distal muscles.[64,116,117] Repetitive studies are less likely to be abnormal than in MuSK antibody-negative patients.[65,118] Single fiber electromyography is usually abnormal in the facial muscles, but less likely to be abnormal in the limbs.[68,118,119] Electromyography findings often show severe myopathic changes with reduced amplitude and duration without polyphasia in affected muscles.[116,120–122] Fibrillation potentials are reported more frequently than in AChR antibody-positive MG.[116] In our patient, increased insertional activity was seen, and only a few very small units were seen in the orbicularis oculi. Muscle atrophy, particularly in the face and tongue midline, atrophy are very prevalent in these patients[105,123–125]; however, some series found tongue atrophy to be uncommon.[78,108,116] Muscle biopsies from patients with MuSK antibody-positive MG have severe myopathic and mitochondrial abnormalities.[126,127] MRI studies have shown that facial muscle bulk is less in abnormal patients.[123,128] After successful treatment, previously seen tongue atrophy improves in MuSK antibody-positive MG.[76,129] The increased atrophy preferentially seen in the facial muscles compared with limb muscles might be related to reduced levels of MuSK found in facial and respiratory muscles.[130,131] The type of immunoglobulins causing MuSK antibody-positive MG might play a role in the differences in the clinical course. Unlike AChR antibody-positive MG, where IgG1 and IgG3 antibodies cause complement activation, IgG4 antibodies are found in MuSK antibody-positive MG.[132–134] It is believed that IgG4 antibodies may block MuSK signaling by interfering with the binding of LRP4 to MuSK, thereby destabilizing the neuromuscular junction.[132,133,135,136]

Treatment of MuSK antibody-positive MG differs somewhat from AChR antibody-positive MG. Patients with MuSK antibody-positive MG tend to respond less to pyridostigmine and other cholinesterase inhibitors.[78,137,138] There have been reports of worsening of symptoms with pyridostigmine in MuSK antibody-positive MG.[79] These patients respond less often and have a lower tolerance to cholinesterase inhibitors with more nicotinic and muscarinic side effects.[138] One explanation for this finding is that COLQ, which binds acetylcholinesterase to the neuromuscular junction, is also bound to MuSK and antibodies to MuSK might affect this connection.[133,139] These interactions might impair acetylcholinesterase activity at baseline in MuSK antibody-positive MG and further interference by cholinesterase inhibitors might produce worsening symptoms. In a mouse model of MuSK antibody-positive MG, 3,4-diaminopyridine has been shown to be efficacious.[140] In addition, 3,4-diaminopyridine, which enhances the release of acetylcholine from the axonal terminal, has been shown to be of benefit in patients with MuSK antibody-positive MG.[141] This is due to 3,4-diaminopyridine increasing the amount of acetylcholine in the neuromuscular junction rather than increasing its duration of action as pyridostigmine would.[142] Generally, pyridostigmine should be tried at a low dose initially in patients with MuSK antibody-positive MG, but its actions need to be monitored, because it is often not beneficial and could worsen symptoms. If not beneficial at 90 mg every 4 hours, no further dose escalation should be considered. If available, 3,4-diaminopyridine might be considered as an alternative treatment.

In most instances, patients respond to immunosuppressant therapy. Prednisone, azathioprine, mycophenolate, tacrolimus, methotrexate, and cyclosporine have been tried with success in these patients.[64,78,80,116,126,143,144] The initial therapy would include prednisone combined with a steroid sparing immunosuppressant. Prednisone should be started at a dose of 40 to 60 mg/d and decreased to the lowest effective dose. In most instances, these patients respond similarly to patients with AChR antibody-positive MG. For acute exacerbations of MuSK antibody-positive MG, intravenous immunoglobulin, and plasma exchange have been used, but intravenous immunoglobulin is less efficacious than plasma exchange in most patients.[63,78,80,145] On occasion patients, will respond to intravenous immunoglobulin who have not responded well to plasma exchange, but this is less common.[126,146,147] Patients with poorly responsive disease have responded well to rituximab 375 mg/m², weekly for 4 weeks. Often the response to rituximab is better than what is seen in AChR antibody-positive MG and can lead to long-lasting remissions lasting 6 months to longer than a year. There is a report of a patient responding to high-dose cyclophosphamide at 50 mg/kg for 4 days who had failed other therapies, including rituximab.[148] There have also been reports of patients going into spontaneous remission.[149]

In summary, although many cases of MuSK antibody-positive MG present with distinct symptoms consisting of bulbar, facial, and respiratory weakness and may have a more severe course of the disease, other patients present with head drop or with symptoms typical of AChR antibody-positive MG. In most patients with MuSK antibody-positive MG, with proper immunosuppressant therapy, symptoms can be well-controlled.[78]

LOW-DENSITY LIPOPROTEIN RECEPTOR-RELATED PROTEIN 4 ANTIBODY-POSITIVE MYASTHENIA GRAVIS

After the discovery of MuSK antibody-positive MG, around 10% to 13% of patients with MG remain negative (ie, for antibodies against AChR and MuSK, and thus double-negative MG [DNMG]). Since the discovery of LRP4,[36,37] it was felt that it would be a good target for autoimmune attack, because much of this molecule is extracellular. Three groups simultaneously reported the presence of LRP4 antibodies in MG.[10–12] Shen and colleagues[150] showed that mice injected with LRP4 developed weakness, a decremental response to repetitive stimulation, and produced LRP4 antibodies. These antibodies reduced cell-surface LRP4 level, agrin activation of MuSK, and the aggregation of AChR at the neuromuscular junction. Furthermore, these antibodies were predominantly IgG1 followed by IgG2 and IgG3, which are known to activate complement. Using mice that are genetically designed to delete the LRP4 gene when exposed to doxycycline, LRP4 has been shown to be essential to the preservation of the neuromuscular junction.[151] These mice develop weakness and neuromuscular transmission failure. LRP4 also has been shown to have retrograde effects on the axonal terminal producing presynaptic differentiation.[152,153] Since the discovery of LRP4 antibody-positive MG some data have been reported on these patients, but there is only limited information about the characteristics of these patients.

The following case from one of the authors (M.H.R.), illustrates a patient with LRP4 antibody-positive MG. The patient is a 49-year-old white woman who developed shortness of breath, a soft voice, and generalized fatigue 2 years before her first visit. She complained of intermittent facial weakness and fatigue while chewing and periodic difficulty swallowing both liquids and solids. She had ptosis and diplopia. She fatigues, feeling that her weakness is worse in the afternoon. Her AChR, MuSK, and voltage-gated calcium channel antibodies were negative. She had normal repetitive nerve and pulmonary function testing. She is unable to tolerate pyridostigmine because of gastrointestinal side effects. She had a gastric bypass in the past. She had bilateral ptosis with mild diplopia. She had mild weakness of her orbicularis oculi, orbicularis oris, masseter, and sternocleidomastoid muscles. She had mild dysarthria. The remainder of her cranial nerves were normal. She had moderate neck weakness. She had mild proximal arm weakness. Needle examination of her right deltoid was normal. Single fiber electromyography of her orbicularis oculi was abnormal with 50% of her fibers having increased jitter and 8% showing block. Left biceps muscle biopsy showed mild type II atrophy. Her LRP4 antibody level is 0.471 (normal, <0.267). Her agrin antibody level is also elevated at 0.446 (normal, <0.264). She is on prednisone, methotrexate, and azathioprine, and is uncertain of improvement. She responds very well to plasma exchange, noting an improvement in strength after every treatment. She recently received a course of rituximab, but it is too early to know if she received benefit. When weakest she was MGFA class[81] IIIb.

In most cases described in the literature, LRP4 antibodies are more common in women than men.[154] The prevalence in DNMG has been as low as 2% to 4% in Asian populations[10,155] to as high as 53% in a study from Pevzner and colleagues.[11] In the largest reported series, Zisimopoulou and colleagues[154] found a prevalence of 18.7%. Regional variation in prevalence has been reported.[154] Most cases are described as mild to moderate, and the ocular muscles are usually involved.[154–156] Despite this, some patients have more severe symptoms (classes III and IV).[10,11,154] Patients having myasthenic crises have been described (class V).[10,11,154,157] Patients with antibodies for both LRP4 and AChR or MuSK are more symptomatic and do less well than patients with only LRP4 antibodies.[154,156] One of our patients with LRP4 antibodies had voltage-gated calcium channel antibodies and has features of both MG and Lambert Eaton myasthenic syndrome. Currently, these patients generally present similarly to patients with AChR antibody-positive MG, but their symptoms are usually milder. Most patients respond to pyridostigmine, steroids, and immunosuppressant medications like other patients with MG. Thymus pathology is usually not present, but has been described, including thymomas.[154,155,158] Although in most cases respiratory dysfunction is mild, respiratory failure has been described.[157]

LRP4 is an important signaling receptor in many other systems and is important for development. LRP4 antibodies have not been seen in control patients with other diseases, except in 10% of patients with amyotrophic lateral sclerosis[159,160] and 2 cases of neuromyelitis optica.[12] Whether it is pathogenic in amyotrophic lateral sclerosis is not currently known. Because LRP4 antibodies are present in approximately 13% to 18% of patients with DNMG and LRP4 antibodies have been shown to produce pathology in mice, it could in the future be part of routine MG patient screening. Further research is needed to understand what features are seen in these patients and determine its prevalence.

AGRIN AND OTHER ANTIBODIES IN MYASTHENIA GRAVIS

Agrin is another potential target for antibodies that can produce MG. Four papers found agrin antibodies in patients with MG.[13,14,156,161] In these studies, most of the patients are positive for other antibodies as well.[13,14,156,161] Four of the patients reported by Gasperi and associates,[13] but none of the patients reported by Cossins and coworkers,[161] Zhang and colleagues,[14] or Cordts and coworkers[156] had antibodies to MuSK. In all 4 studies, patients with agrin-positive MG had antibodies to AChR as well: 13 reported by Cossins and colleagues,[161] 1 reported by Gasperi and cowrkers,[13] 5 reported by Zhang and associates,[14] and 3 reported by Cordts and associates.[156] In addition, 1 patient who was positive for agrin and MuSK antibodies also had antibodies to LRP4.[13] There is a total of 14 patients reported who have antibodies only to agrin, but clinical data were available for only 1 patient.[14,156,161] This patient was MGFA class III and only partially responded to pyridostigmine and prednisone.[156] Based on these limited data, the incidence and clinical characteristics of patients with agrin antibody-positive MG are unknown. Further research is required before we can know the role of agrin antibodies in MG. Perhaps the coexistence of these antibodies might have implications on the severity of the disease. Similar to LRP4 antibodies, agrin antibodies have been seen in patients with amyotrophic lateral sclerosis, even though their role is unknown in this disease state.[159]

Titin is a large structural protein found in muscle that extends the entire length of the sarcomere and has an important role in muscle elasticity. Although this protein is very large, antibodies are directed against a small segment at the A/I band junction, representing less than 1% of this protein. These antibodies have been found in patients with MG, often in association with other pathogenic antibodies.[16] Titin antibodies are age related, often being found in older patients with MG. These antibodies have been associated with thymoma in thymectomized patients[16] and may have predictive value in determining which patients have thymomas. More recently, 2 studies looked at titin antibodies in seronegative MG.[15,156] Cordts and colleagues[156] found that 23% of seronegative MG had titin antibodies, whereas Stergiou and colleagues[15] found that 18% were positive. In both studies, patients positive for only titin antibodies have milder disease and are responsive to therapy. Patients with AChR and titin antibodies have more severe disease and are more likely to have thymomas. Further research is needed to determine if this antibody is causative or just a bystander antibody.

Agius and colleagues[18] describe rapsyn antibodies in patients with MG. This substance was found in around 13% of the limited number of patients tested. However, these antibodies were nonspecific and are of uncertain significance. Congenital defects in rapsyn are associated with congenital MG.[21,22,25] Antibodies to ColQ have been found in 6 patients with MG (4%), of which 4 patients had DNMG.[161] The significance of these antibodies is unknown.

Gallardo and colleagues[17] describes antibodies to cortactin in 19.7% of 91 patients with DNMG. These antibodies were found in only 4.8% of either AChR antibody-positive or MuSK antibody-positive patients. None of these patients were positive for LRP4. These patients were predominantly women (68%) and most were less than 50 years old at disease onset. Twenty-two percent had ocular disease and the remainder had generalized disease with ocular predominance. One patient had a thymoma. Cortactin antibodies are also detected in 12.5% of patients with other autoimmune neurologic diseases. In a study of 250 MG cases, most had AChR antibodies, 11 had MuSK antibodies, and 28 had antibodies to cortactin.[162] Of those, only 9 were DNMG and most[19] had AChR antibodies. The frequency of cortactin antibodies was significantly higher in the DNMG group (23.7%) compared with the AChR-positive group (9.5%). No patients in this study had antibodies to both cortactin and MuSK. The 9 DNMG cortactin antibody–positive patients had either ocular MG or mild MG (MGFA grade IIA) and fewer bulbar symptoms. Of 17 patients with ocular DNMG, 23.5% had antibodies to cortactin. The role of these antibodies remains unknown and requires further study.

SUMMARY

New antigenic targets have been discovered that might account for many of the AChR antibody-negative patients with MG. The best studied of these is anti-MuSK antibody MG. In some instances, their distinctive phenotype might raise the clinical suspicion for this form of the disease. Treatment of these patients is similar to that of AChR antibody-positive MG, with the notable exception that they are less responsive to cholinesterase inhibitors such as pyridostigmine. In addition, difficult-to-treat patients with MuSK antibody-positive MG generally have an excellent response to rituximab. Antistriatal muscle antibodies seen in one-third of MG cases are nonspecific to MG and are not a reliable predictor of thymic pathology. Although there is less experience with LRP4 antibody-positive MG, there is evidence that antibodies to LRP4 can cause neuromuscular defects. At this point, there are no specific phenotypes for this form of MG, but it usually causes a milder form of the disease even though there are notable exceptions. Treatment for these patients is like that of patients with AChR antibody-positive disease. The role of agrin, titin, and cortactin antibodies are currently unknown and more research is needed. These antibodies are associated with the disease, but we do not know if they cause the disease or are an epiphenomenon. With more information about the role of these antibodies, we might be able to diagnose patient with MG earlier and design better therapies.

DISCLOSURE STATEMENT

Dr M.H. Rivner is on the speaker's bureau for Allergan and has received grants from Allergan, Alexion, Biogen, Cytokinetics, Elan, GlaxoSmithKline, Grifols, and UCB. Dr M. Pasnoo has no disclosures to make. Dr M. Dimachkie is on the speaker's bureau or is a consultant for Alnylam, Baxalta, Catalyst, CSL-Behring, Mallinckrodt, Novartis, and NuFactor. He has also received grants from Alexion, Biomarin, Catalyst, CSL Behring, FDA/OPD, GSK, Grifols, MDA, National Institutes of Health, Novartis, Sanofi, and TMA. Dr R. Barohn is on the speaker's bureau for NuFactor, Grifols Therapeutics Inc, and Plan 365 Inc. He is on the advisory board for CSL Behring GmbH, and has received an honorarium from Option Care. He has received research grants from National Institutes of Health, FDA/OOPD, NINDS, Novartis, Sanofi/Genzyme, Biomarin, IONIS, Teva, Cytokinetics, Eli Lilly, and PTC. Dr L. Mei has a patent with Augusta University on a LRP4 assay. He has received grants from the National Institutes of Health and the Veterans Administration. This work was supported by a CTSA grant from

NCATS awarded to the University of Kansas for Frontiers: University of Kansas Clinical and Translational Science Institute (# UL1TR002366) The contents are solely the responsibility of the authors and do not necessarily represent the official views of the NIH or NCATS.

REFERENCES

1. Lindstrom JM, Seybold ME, Lennon VA, et al. Antibody to acetylcholine receptor in myasthenia gravis. Prevalence, clinical correlates, and diagnostic value. Neurology 1976;26(11):1054–9.
2. Evoli A, Batocchi AP, Lo Monaco M, et al. Clinical heterogeneity of seronegative myasthenia gravis. Neuromuscul Disord 1996;6(3):155–61.
3. Birmanns B, Brenner T, Abramsky O, et al. Seronegative myasthenia gravis: clinical features, response to therapy and synthesis of acetylcholine receptor antibodies in vitro. J Neurol Sci 1991;102(2):184–9.
4. Mossman S, Vincent A, Newsom-Davis J. Myasthenia gravis without acetylcholine-receptor antibody: a distinct disease entity. Lancet 1986; 1(8473):116–9.
5. Oteiza Orradre C, Navarro Serrano E, Rebage Moises V, et al. Seronegative transient neonatal myasthenia: report of a case. An Esp Pediatr 1996;45(6): 651–2 [in Spanish].
6. Sisman J, Ceri A, Nafday SM. Seronegative neonatal myasthenia gravis in one of the twins. Indian Pediatr 2004;41(9):938–40.
7. Townsel C, Keller R, Johnson K, et al. Seronegative maternal ocular myasthenia gravis and delayed transient neonatal myasthenia gravis. AJP Rep 2016;6(1): e133–6.
8. Blaes F, Beeson D, Plested P, et al. IgG from "seronegative" myasthenia gravis patients binds to a muscle cell line, TE671, but not to human acetylcholine receptor. Ann Neurol 2000;47(4):504–10.
9. Hoch W, McConville J, Helms S, et al. Auto-antibodies to the receptor tyrosine kinase MuSK in patients with myasthenia gravis without acetylcholine receptor antibodies. Nat Med 2001;7(3):365–8.
10. Higuchi O, Hamuro J, Motomura M, et al. Autoantibodies to low-density lipoprotein receptor-related protein 4 in myasthenia gravis. Ann Neurol 2011;69(2): 418–22.
11. Pevzner A, Schoser B, Peters K, et al. Anti-LRP4 autoantibodies in AChR- and MuSK-antibody-negative myasthenia gravis. J Neurol 2012;259(3):427–35.
12. Zhang B, Tzartos JS, Belimezi M, et al. Autoantibodies to lipoprotein-related protein 4 in patients with double-seronegative myasthenia gravis. Arch Neurol 2012;69(4):445–51.
13. Gasperi C, Melms A, Schoser B, et al. Anti-agrin autoantibodies in myasthenia gravis. Neurology 2014;82(22):1976–83.
14. Zhang B, Shen C, Bealmear B, et al. Autoantibodies to agrin in myasthenia gravis patients. PLoS One 2014;9(3):e91816.
15. Stergiou C, Lazaridis K, Zouvelou V, et al. Titin antibodies in "seronegative" myasthenia gravis–a new role for an old antigen. J Neuroimmunol 2016;292: 108–15.
16. Yamamoto AM, Gajdos P, Eymard B, et al. Anti-titin antibodies in myasthenia gravis: tight association with thymoma and heterogeneity of nonthymoma patients. Arch Neurol 2001;58(6):885–90.

17. Gallardo E, Martinez-Hernandez E, Titulaer MJ, et al. Cortactin autoantibodies in myasthenia gravis. Autoimmun Rev 2014;13(10):1003–7.
18. Agius MA, Zhu S, Kirvan CA, et al. Rapsyn antibodies in myasthenia gravis. Ann N Y Acad Sci 1998;841:516–21.
19. Bogdanik LP, Burgess RW. A valid mouse model of AGRIN-associated congenital myasthenic syndrome. Hum Mol Genet 2011;20(23):4617–33.
20. Huze C, Bauche S, Richard P, et al. Identification of an agrin mutation that causes congenital myasthenia and affects synapse function. Am J Hum Genet 2009;85(2):155–67.
21. Burke G, Cossins J, Maxwell S, et al. Rapsyn mutations in hereditary myasthenia: distinct early- and late-onset phenotypes. Neurology 2003;61(6):826–8.
22. Dunne V, Maselli RA. Identification of pathogenic mutations in the human rapsyn gene. J Hum Genet 2003;48(4):204–7.
23. Ioos C, Barois A, Richard P, et al. Congenital myasthenic syndrome due to rapsyn deficiency: three cases with arthrogryposis and bulbar symptoms. Neuropediatrics 2004;35(4):246–9.
24. Maselli R, Dris H, Schnier J, et al. Congenital myasthenic syndrome caused by two non-N88K rapsyn mutations. Clin Genet 2007;72(1):63–5.
25. Maselli RA, Dunne V, Pascual-Pascual SI, et al. Rapsyn mutations in myasthenic syndrome due to impaired receptor clustering. Muscle Nerve 2003;28(3):293–301.
26. Muller JS, Mildner G, Muller-Felber W, et al. Rapsyn N88K is a frequent cause of congenital myasthenic syndromes in European patients. Neurology 2003;60(11):1805–10.
27. Ohno K, Engel AG, Shen XM, et al. Rapsyn mutations in humans cause endplate acetylcholine-receptor deficiency and myasthenic syndrome. Am J Hum Genet 2002;70(4):875–85.
28. Ben Ammar A, Soltanzadeh P, Bauche S, et al. A mutation causes MuSK reduced sensitivity to agrin and congenital myasthenia. PLoS One 2013;8(1):e53826.
29. Luan X, Tian W, Cao L. Limb-girdle congenital myasthenic syndrome in a Chinese family with novel mutations in MUSK gene and literature review. Clin Neurol Neurosurg 2016;150:41–5.
30. Maselli RA, Arredondo J, Cagney O, et al. Mutations in MUSK causing congenital myasthenic syndrome impair MuSK-Dok-7 interaction. Hum Mol Genet 2010;19(12):2370–9.
31. Selcen D, Ohkawara B, Shen XM, et al. Impaired synaptic development, maintenance, and neuromuscular transmission in LRP4-related myasthenia. JAMA Neurol 2015;72(8):889–96.
32. Maselli RA, Fernandez JM, Arredondo J, et al. LG2 agrin mutation causing severe congenital myasthenic syndrome mimics functional characteristics of non-neural (z-) agrin. Hum Genet 2012;131(7):1123–35.
33. Nicole S, Chaouch A, Torbergsen T, et al. Agrin mutations lead to a congenital myasthenic syndrome with distal muscle weakness and atrophy. Brain 2014;137(Pt 9):2429–43.
34. Ohkawara B, Cabrera-Serrano M, Nakata T, et al. LRP4 third beta-propeller domain mutations cause novel congenital myasthenia by compromising agrin-mediated MuSK signaling in a position-specific manner. Hum Mol Genet 2014;23(7):1856–68.
35. Tsen G, Halfter W, Kroger S, et al. Agrin is a heparan sulfate proteoglycan. J Biol Chem 1995;270(7):3392–9.

36. Kim N, Stiegler AL, Cameron TO, et al. Lrp4 is a receptor for Agrin and forms a complex with MuSK. Cell 2008;135(2):334–42.

37. Zhang B, Luo S, Wang Q, et al. LRP4 serves as a coreceptor of agrin. Neuron 2008;60(2):285–97.

38. Dimitropoulou A, Bixby JL. Motor neurite outgrowth is selectively inhibited by cell surface MuSK and Agrin. Mol Cell Neurosci 2005;28(2):292–302.

39. Cartaud A, Strochlic L, Guerra M, et al. MuSK is required for anchoring acetylcholinesterase at the neuromuscular junction. J Cell Biol 2004;165(4):505–15.

40. Karmouch J, Dobbertin A, Sigoillot S, et al. Developmental consequences of the ColQ/MuSK interactions. Chem Biol Interact 2013;203(1):287–91.

41. Nakata T, Ito M, Azuma Y, et al. Mutations in the C-terminal domain of ColQ in endplate acetylcholinesterase deficiency compromise ColQ-MuSK interaction. Hum Mutat 2013;34(7):997–1004.

42. Zong Y, Zhang B, Gu S, et al. Structural basis of agrin-LRP4-MuSK signaling. Genes Dev 2012;26(3):247–58.

43. Bergamin E, Hallock PT, Burden SJ, et al. The cytoplasmic adaptor protein Dok7 activates the receptor tyrosine kinase MuSK via dimerization. Mol Cell 2010; 39(1):100–9.

44. Ueta R, Tezuka T, Izawa Y, et al. The carboxyl-terminal region of Dok-7 plays a key, but not essential, role in activation of muscle-specific receptor kinase MuSK and neuromuscular synapse formation. J Biochem 2017;161(3):269–77.

45. Inoue A, Setoguchi K, Matsubara Y, et al. Dok-7 activates the muscle receptor kinase MuSK and shapes synapse formation. Sci Signal 2009;2(59):ra7.

46. Yamanashi Y, Higuch O, Beeson D. Dok-7/MuSK signaling and a congenital myasthenic syndrome. Acta Myol 2008;27:25–9.

47. Antolik C, Catino DH, Resneck WG, et al. The tetratricopeptide repeat domains of rapsyn bind directly to cytoplasmic sequences of the muscle-specific kinase. Neuroscience 2006;141(1):87–100.

48. Apel ED, Glass DJ, Moscoso LM, et al. Rapsyn is required for MuSK signaling and recruits synaptic components to a MuSK-containing scaffold. Neuron 1997; 18(4):623–35.

49. Frail DE, McLaughlin LL, Mudd J, et al. Identification of the mouse muscle 43,000-dalton acetylcholine receptor-associated protein (RAPsyn) by cDNA cloning. J Biol Chem 1988;263(30):15602–7.

50. Gautam M, Noakes PG, Mudd J, et al. Failure of postsynaptic specialization to develop at neuromuscular junctions of rapsyn-deficient mice. Nature 1995; 377(6546):232–6.

51. Lee Y, Rudell J, Ferns M. Rapsyn interacts with the muscle acetylcholine receptor via alpha-helical domains in the alpha, beta, and epsilon subunit intracellular loops. Neuroscience 2009;163(1):222–32.

52. Zuber B, Unwin N. Structure and superorganization of acetylcholine receptor-rapsyn complexes. Proc Natl Acad Sci U S A 2013;110(26):10622–7.

53. Burden SJ, DePalma RL, Gottesman GS. Crosslinking of proteins in acetylcholine receptor-rich membranes: association between the beta-subunit and the 43 kd subsynaptic protein. Cell 1983;35(3 Pt 2):687–92.

54. Bartoli M, Ramarao MK, Cohen JB. Interactions of the rapsyn RING-H2 domain with dystroglycan. J Biol Chem 2001;276(27):24911–7.

55. Valenzuela DM, Stitt TN, DiStefano PS, et al. Receptor tyrosine kinase specific for the skeletal muscle lineage: expression in embryonic muscle, at the neuromuscular junction, and after injury. Neuron 1995;15(3):573–84.

56. DeChiara TM, Bowen DC, Valenzuela DM, et al. The receptor tyrosine kinase MuSK is required for neuromuscular junction formation in vivo. Cell 1996; 85(4):501–12.
57. Glass DJ, Bowen DC, Stitt TN, et al. Agrin acts via a MuSK receptor complex. Cell 1996;85(4):513–23.
58. Cole RN, Reddel SW, Gervasio OL, et al. Anti-MuSK patient antibodies disrupt the mouse neuromuscular junction. Ann Neurol 2008;63(6):782–9.
59. Jha S, Xu K, Maruta T, et al. Myasthenia gravis induced in mice by immunization with the recombinant extracellular domain of rat muscle-specific kinase (MuSK). J Neuroimmunol 2006;175(1–2):107–17.
60. Benveniste O, Jacobson L, Farrugia ME, et al. MuSK antibody positive myasthenia gravis plasma modifies MURF-1 expression in C2C12 cultures and mouse muscle in vivo. J Neuroimmunol 2005;170(1–2):41–8.
61. Lee JY, Sung JJ, Cho JY, et al. MuSK antibody-positive, seronegative myasthenia gravis in Korea. J Clin Neurosci 2006;13(3):353–5.
62. Chan KH, Lachance DH, Harper CM, et al. Frequency of seronegativity in adult-acquired generalized myasthenia gravis. Muscle Nerve 2007;36(5):651–8.
63. Sanders DB, El-Salem K, Massey JM, et al. Clinical aspects of MuSK antibody positive seronegative MG. Neurology 2003;60(12):1978–80.
64. Evoli A, Tonali PA, Padua L, et al. Clinical correlates with anti-MuSK antibodies in generalized seronegative myasthenia gravis. Brain 2003;126:2304–11.
65. Padua L, Tonali P, Aprile I, et al. Seronegative myasthenia gravis: comparison of neurophysiological picture in MuSK+ and MuSK-patients. Eur J Neurol 2006; 13(3):273–6.
66. Hurst RL, Gooch CL. Muscle-specific receptor tyrosine kinase (MuSK) myasthenia gravis. Curr Neurol Neurosci Rep 2016;16(7):61.
67. Lavrnic D, Losen M, Vujic A, et al. The features of myasthenia gravis with auto-antibodies to MuSK. J Neurol Neurosurg Psychiatry 2005;76(8):1099–102.
68. Stickler DE, Massey JM, Sanders DB. MuSK-antibody positive myasthenia gravis: clinical and electrodiagnostic patterns. Clin Neurophysiol 2005;116(9): 2065–8.
69. Huang YC, Yeh JH, Chiu HC, et al. Clinical characteristics of MuSK antibody-positive myasthenia gravis in Taiwan. J Formos Med Assoc 2008;107(7):572–5.
70. Yeh JH, Chen WH, Chiu HC, et al. Low frequency of MuSK antibody in generalized seronegative myasthenia gravis among Chinese. Neurology 2004;62(11): 2131–2.
71. Kostera-Pruszczyk A, Kaminska A, Dutkiewicz M, et al. MuSK-positive myasthenia gravis is rare in the Polish population. Eur J Neurol 2008;15(7):720–4.
72. Bartoccioni E, Scuderi F, Augugliaro A, et al. HLA class II allele analysis in MuSK-positive myasthenia gravis suggests a role for DQ5. Neurology 2009; 72(2):195–7.
73. Alahgholi-Hajibehzad M, Yilmaz V, Gulsen-Parman Y, et al. Association of HLA-DRB1*14, -DRB1 *16 and -DQB1 *05 with MuSK-myasthenia gravis in patients from Turkey. Hum Immunol 2013;74(12):1633–5.
74. Kanai T, Uzawa A, Kawaguchi N, et al. HLA-DRB1*14 and DQB1*05 are associated with Japanese anti-MuSK antibody-positive myasthenia gravis patients. J Neurol Sci 2016;363:116–8.
75. Furuta N, Ishizawa K, Shibata M, et al. Anti-MuSK antibody-positive myasthenia gravis mimicking amyotrophic lateral sclerosis. Intern Med 2015;54(19): 2497–501.

76. Takahashi H, Kawaguchi N, Ito S, et al. Is tongue atrophy reversible in anti-MuSK myasthenia gravis? Six-year observation. J Neurol Neurosurg Psychiatry 2010; 81(6):701–2.

77. Ohno K, Ito M, Kawakami Y, et al. Collagen Q is a key player for developing rational therapy for congenital myasthenia and for dissecting the mechanisms of anti-MuSK myasthenia gravis. J Mol Neurosci 2014;53(3):359–61.

78. Pasnoor M, Wolfe GI, Nations S, et al. Clinical findings in MuSK-antibody positive myasthenia gravis: a U.S. experience. Muscle Nerve 2010;41(3):370–4.

79. Punga AR, Flink R, Askmark H, et al. Cholinergic neuromuscular hyperactivity in patients with myasthenia gravis seropositive for MuSK antibody. Muscle Nerve 2006;34(1):111–5.

80. Evoli A, Bianchi MR, Riso R, et al. Response to therapy in myasthenia gravis with anti-MuSK antibodies. Ann N Y Acad Sci 2008;1132:76–83.

81. Jaretzki A, Barohn RJ, Ernstoff RM, et al. Myasthenia gravis: recommendations for clinical research standards. Neurology 2000;55(1):16–23.

82. Caress JB, Hunt CH, Batish SD. Anti-MuSK myasthenia gravis presenting with purely ocular findings. Arch Neurol 2005;62(6):1002–3.

83. Bau V, Hanisch F, Hain B, et al. Ocular involvement in MuSK antibody-positive myasthenia gravis. Klin Monbl Augenheilkd 2006;223(1):81–3 [in German].

84. Bennett DL, Mills KR, Riordan-Eva P, et al. Anti-MuSK antibodies in a case of ocular myasthenia gravis. J Neurol Neurosurg Psychiatry 2006;77(4):564–5.

85. Chan JW, Orrison WW. Ocular myasthenia: a rare presentation with MuSK antibody and bilateral extraocular muscle atrophy. Br J Ophthalmol 2007;91(6): 842–3.

86. Hanisch F, Eger K, Zierz S. MuSK-antibody positive pure ocular myasthenia gravis. J Neurol 2006;253(5):659–60.

87. Hosaka A, Takuma H, Ohta K, et al. An ocular form of myasthenia gravis with a high titer of anti-MuSK antibodies during a long-term follow-up. Intern Med 2012;51(21):3077–9.

88. Casasnovas C, Povedano M, Jauma S, et al. Musk-antibody positive myasthenia gravis presenting with isolated neck extensor weakness. Neuromuscul Disord 2007;17(7):544–6.

89. Okano T, Fujitake J, Suzuki K, et al. A case of anti-MuSK antibody-positive myasthenia gravis with dropped head as the initial presenting symptom. Rinsho Shinkeigaku 2006;46(7):496–500 [in Japanese].

90. Spengos K, Vassilopoulou S, Papadimas G, et al. Dropped head syndrome as prominent clinical feature in MuSK-positive Myasthenia Gravis with thymus hyperplasia. Neuromuscul Disord 2008;18(2):175–7.

91. Giarrana ML, Joset P, Sticht H, et al. A severe congenital myasthenic syndrome with "dropped head" caused by novel MUSK mutations. Muscle Nerve 2015; 52(4):668–73.

92. Hara K, Mashima T, Matsuda A, et al. Vocal cord paralysis in myasthenia gravis with anti-MuSK antibodies. Neurology 2007;68(8):621–2.

93. Jimenez Caballero PE, Fermin Marrero JA, Trigo Bragado I, et al. Vocal cord paralysis as a manifestation of myasthenia gravis with anti-MuSK antibodies. Neurologia 2014;29(4):253–4.

94. Sylva M, van der Kooi AJ, Grolman W. Dyspnoea due to vocal fold abduction paresis in anti-MuSK myasthenia gravis. J Neurol Neurosurg Psychiatry 2008; 79(9):1083–4.

95. Zouvelou V, Kyriazi S, Rentzos M, et al. Double-seropositive myasthenia gravis. Muscle Nerve 2013;47(3):465–6.

96. Zouvelou V, Zisimopoulou P, Psimenou E, et al. AChR-myasthenia gravis switching to double-seropositive several years after the onset. J Neuroimmunol 2014; 267(1–2):111–2.
97. Basta I, Nikolic A, Losen M, et al. MuSK myasthenia gravis and Lambert-Eaton myasthenic syndrome in the same patient. Clin Neurol Neurosurg 2012;114(6): 795–7.
98. Diaz-Manera J, Rojas-Garcia R, Gallardo E, et al. Antibodies to AChR, MuSK and VGKC in a patient with myasthenia gravis and Morvan's syndrome. Nat Clin Pract Neurol 2007;3(7):405–10.
99. Bartoccioni E, Scuderi F, Minicuci GM, et al. Anti-MuSK antibodies: correlation with myasthenia gravis severity. Neurology 2006;67(3):505–7.
100. Behin A, Mayer M, Kassis-Makhoul B, et al. Severe neonatal myasthenia due to maternal anti-MuSK antibodies. Neuromuscul Disord 2008;18(6):443–6.
101. Kanzaki A, Motomura M. A pregnant patient with anti-MuSK antibody positive myasthenia gravis and her infant with transient neonatal myasthenia gravis. Rinsho Shinkeigaku 2011;51(3):188–91 [in Japanese].
102. Murray EL, Kedar S, Vedanarayanan VV. Transmission of maternal muscle-specific tyrosine kinase (MuSK) to offspring: report of two cases. J Clin Neuromuscul Dis 2010;12(2):76–9.
103. Niks EH, Verrips A, Semmekrot BA, et al. A transient neonatal myasthenic syndrome with anti-musk antibodies. Neurology 2008;70(14):1215–6.
104. O'Carroll P, Bertorini TE, Jacob G, et al. Transient neonatal myasthenia gravis in a baby born to a mother with new-onset anti-MuSK-mediated myasthenia gravis. J Clin Neuromuscul Dis 2009;11(2):69–71.
105. Guptill JT, Sanders DB. Update on muscle-specific tyrosine kinase antibody positive myasthenia gravis. Curr Opin Neurol 2010;23(5):530–5.
106. Saka E, Topcuoglu MA, Akkaya B, et al. Thymus changes in anti-MuSK-positive and -negative myasthenia gravis. Neurology 2005;65(5):782–3 [author reply: 782–3].
107. Ito A, Sasaki R, Ii Y, et al. A case of thymoma-associated myasthenia gravis with anti-MuSK antibodies. Rinsho Shinkeigaku 2013;53(5):372–5 [in Japanese].
108. Tsonis AI, Zisimopoulou P, Lazaridis K, et al. MuSK autoantibodies in myasthenia gravis detected by cell based assay–a multinational study. J Neuroimmunol 2015;284:10–7.
109. Lauriola L, Ranelletti F, Maggiano N, et al. Thymus changes in anti-MuSK-positive and -negative myasthenia gravis. Neurology 2005;64(3):536–8.
110. Leite MI, Strobel P, Jones M, et al. Fewer thymic changes in MuSK antibody-positive than in MuSK antibody-negative MG. Ann Neurol 2005;57(3):444–8.
111. Ponseti JM, Caritg N, Gamez J, et al. A comparison of long-term post-thymectomy outcome of anti-AChR-positive, anti-AChR-negative and anti-MuSK-positive patients with non-thymomatous myasthenia gravis. Expert Opin Biol Ther 2009;9(1):1–8.
112. Kostera-Pruszczyk A, Kwiecinski H. Juvenile seropositive myasthenia gravis with anti-MuSK antibody after thymectomy. J Neurol 2009;256(10):1780–1.
113. Saulat B, Maertens P, Hamilton WJ, et al. Anti-musk antibody after thymectomy in a previously seropositive myasthenic child. Neurology 2007;69(8):803–4.
114. Jordan B, Schilling S, Zierz S. Switch to double positive late onset MuSK myasthenia gravis following thymomectomy in paraneoplastic AChR antibody positive myasthenia gravis. J Neurol 2016;263(1):174–6.
115. Rajakulendran S, Viegas S, Spillane J, et al. Clinically biphasic myasthenia gravis with both AChR and MuSK antibodies. J Neurol 2012;259(12):2736–9.

116. Oh S. Muscle-specific receptor tyrosine kinase antibody positive myasthenia gravis current status. J Clin Neurol 2009;5:53–64.
117. Oh SJ, Hatanaka Y, Hemmi S, et al. Repetitive nerve stimulation of facial muscles in MuSK antibody-positive myasthenia gravis. Muscle Nerve 2006;33(4):500–4.
118. Nikolic A, Basta I, Stojanovic VR, et al. Electrophysiological profile of the patients with MuSK positive myasthenia gravis. Neurol Res 2014;36(11):945–9.
119. Kuwabara S, Nemoto Y, Misawa S, et al. Anti-MuSK-positive myasthenia gravis: neuromuscular transmission failure in facial and limb muscles. Acta Neurol Scand 2007;115(2):126–8.
120. Farrugia ME, Kennett RP, Hilton-Jones D, et al. Quantitative EMG of facial muscles in myasthenia patients with MuSK antibodies. Clin Neurophysiol 2007; 118(2):269–77.
121. Nikolic A, Basta I, Stojanovic VR, et al. Myopathic changes detected by quantitative electromyography in patients with MuSK and AChR positive myasthenia gravis. J Clin Neurosci 2016;27:126–9.
122. Nikolic AV, Bacic GG, Dakovic MZ, et al. Myopathy, muscle atrophy and tongue lipid composition in MuSK myasthenia gravis. Acta Neurol Belg 2015;115(3): 361–5.
123. Farrugia ME, Robson MD, Clover L, et al. MRI and clinical studies of facial and bulbar muscle involvement in MuSK antibody-associated myasthenia gravis. Brain 2006;129(Pt 6):1481–92.
124. Ishii W, Matsuda M, Okamoto N, et al. Myasthenia gravis with anti-MuSK antibody, showing progressive muscular atrophy without blepharoptosis. Intern Med 2005;44(6):671–2.
125. Moon SY, Lee SS, Hong YH. Muscle atrophy in muscle-specific tyrosine kinase (MuSK)-related myasthenia gravis. J Clin Neurosci 2011;18(9):1274–5.
126. Cenacchi G, Papa V, Fanin M, et al. Comparison of muscle ultrastructure in myasthenia gravis with anti-MuSK and anti-AChR antibodies. J Neurol 2011; 258(5):746–52.
127. Martignago S, Fanin M, Albertini E, et al. Muscle histopathology in myasthenia gravis with antibodies against MuSK and AChR. Neuropathol Appl Neurobiol 2009;35(1):103–10.
128. Zouvelou V, Rentzos M, Toulas P, et al. MRI evidence of early muscle atrophy in MuSK positive myasthenia gravis. J Neuroimaging 2011;21(3):303–5.
129. Kitamura E, Takiyama Y, Nakamura M, et al. Reversible tongue muscle atrophy accelerated by early initiation of immunotherapy in anti-MuSK myasthenia gravis: a case report. J Neurol Sci 2016;360:10–2.
130. Punga AR, Lin S, Oliveri F, et al. Muscle-selective synaptic disassembly and reorganization in MuSK antibody positive MG mice. Exp Neurol 2011;230(2): 207–17.
131. Punga AR, Maj M, Lin S, et al. MuSK levels differ between adult skeletal muscles and influence postsynaptic plasticity. Eur J Neurosci 2011;33(5):890–8.
132. Huijbers MG, Vink AF, Niks EH, et al. Longitudinal epitope mapping in MuSK myasthenia gravis: implications for disease severity. J Neuroimmunol 2016; 291:82–8.
133. Mori S, Shigemoto K. Mechanisms associated with the pathogenicity of antibodies against muscle-specific kinase in myasthenia gravis. Autoimmun Rev 2013;12(9):912–7.
134. Niks EH, van Leeuwen Y, Leite MI, et al. Clinical fluctuations in MuSK myasthenia gravis are related to antigen-specific IgG4 instead of IgG1. J Neuroimmunol 2008;195(1–2):151–6.

135. Huijbers MG, Zhang W, Klooster R, et al. MuSK IgG4 autoantibodies cause myasthenia gravis by inhibiting binding between MuSK and Lrp4. Proc Natl Acad Sci U S A 2013;110(51):20783–8.

136. Koneczny I, Cossins J, Waters P, et al. MuSK myasthenia gravis IgG4 disrupts the interaction of LRP4 with MuSK but both IgG4 and IgG1-3 can disperse pre-formed agrin-independent AChR clusters. PLoS One 2013;8(11):e80695.

137. Hatanaka Y, Hemmi S, Morgan MB, et al. Nonresponsiveness to anticholines-terase agents in patients with MuSK-antibody-positive MG. Neurology 2005; 65(9):1508–9.

138. Shin HY, Park HJ, Lee HE, et al. Clinical and electrophysiologic responses to acetylcholinesterase inhibitors in MuSK-antibody-positive myasthenia gravis: evidence for cholinergic neuromuscular hyperactivity. J Clin Neurol 2014; 10(2):119–24.

139. Plomp JJ, Huijbers MG, van der Maarel SM, et al. Pathogenic IgG4 subclass au-toantibodies in MuSK myasthenia gravis. Ann N Y Acad Sci 2012;1275:114–22.

140. Mori S, Kishi M, Kubo S, et al. 3,4-Diaminopyridine improves neuromuscular transmission in a MuSK antibody-induced mouse model of myasthenia gravis. J Neuroimmunol 2012;245(1–2):75–8.

141. Evoli A, Alboini PE, Damato V, et al. 3,4-Diaminopyridine may improve myas-thenia gravis with MuSK antibodies. Neurology 2016;86(11):1070–1.

142. Morsch M, Reddel SW, Ghazanfari N, et al. Pyridostigmine but not 3,4-diamino-pyridine exacerbates ACh receptor loss and myasthenia induced in mice by muscle-specific kinase autoantibody. J Physiol 2013;591(10):2747–62.

143. El-Salem K, Yassin A, Al-Hayk K, et al. Treatment of MuSK-associated myas-thenia gravis. Curr Treat Options Neurol 2014;16(4):283.

144. Deymeer F, Gungor-Tuncer O, Yilmaz V, et al. Clinical comparison of anti-MuSK-vs anti-AChR-positive and seronegative myasthenia gravis. Neurology 2007; 68(8):609–11.

145. Guptill JT, Sanders DB, Evoli A. Anti-MuSK antibody myasthenia gravis: clinical findings and response to treatment in two large cohorts. Muscle Nerve 2011; 44(1):36–40.

146. Shibata-Hamaguchi A, Samuraki M, Furui E, et al. Long-term effect of intrave-nous immunoglobulin on anti-MuSK antibody-positive myasthenia gravis. Acta Neurol Scand 2007;116(6):406–8.

147. Takahashi H, Kawaguchi N, Nemoto Y, et al. High-dose intravenous immuno-globulin for the treatment of MuSK antibody-positive seronegative myasthenia gravis. J Neurol Sci 2006;247(2):239–41.

148. Lin PT, Martin BA, Weinacker AB, et al. High-dose cyclophosphamide in refrac-tory myasthenia gravis with MuSK antibodies. Muscle Nerve 2006;33(3):433–5.

149. Bouwyn JP, Magnier P, Bedat-Millet AL, et al. Anti-MuSK myasthenia gravis with prolonged remission. Neuromuscul Disord 2016;26(7):453–4.

150. Shen C, Lu Y, Zhang B, et al. Antibodies against low-density lipoprotein receptor-related protein 4 induce myasthenia gravis. J Clin Invest 2013; 123(12):5190–202.

151. Barik A, Lu Y, Sathyamurthy A, et al. LRP4 is critical for neuromuscular junction maintenance. J Neurosci 2014;34(42):13892–905.

152. Yumoto N, Kim N, Burden SJ. Lrp4 is a retrograde signal for presynaptic differ-entiation at neuromuscular synapses. Nature 2012;489(7416):438–42.

153. Wu H, Lu Y, Shen C, et al. Distinct roles of muscle and motoneuron LRP4 in neuromuscular junction formation. Neuron 2012;75(1):94–107.

154. Zisimopoulou P, Evangelakou P, Tzartos J, et al. A comprehensive analysis of the epidemiology and clinical characteristics of anti-LRP4 in myasthenia gravis. J Autoimmun 2014;52:139–45.
155. Li Y, Zhang Y, Cai G, et al. Anti-LRP4 autoantibodies in Chinese patients with myasthenia gravis. Muscle Nerve 2017;56(5):938–42.
156. Cordts I, Bodart N, Hartmann K, et al. Screening for lipoprotein receptor-related protein 4-, agrin-, and titin-antibodies and exploring the autoimmune spectrum in myasthenia gravis. J Neurol 2017;264(6):1193–203.
157. Beck G, Yabumoto T, Baba K, et al. Double seronegative myasthenia gravis with anti-LRP4 antibodies presenting with dropped head and acute respiratory insufficiency. Intern Med 2016;55(22):3361–3.
158. Marino M, Scuderi F, Samengo D, et al. Flow cytofluorimetric analysis of anti-LRP4 (LDL receptor-related protein 4) autoantibodies in Italian patients with myasthenia gravis. PLoS One 2015;10(8):e0135378.
159. Rivner MH, Liu S, Quarles B, et al. Agrin and low-density lipoprotein-related receptor protein 4 antibodies in amyotrophic lateral sclerosis patients. Muscle Nerve 2017;55(3):430–2.
160. Tzartos JS, Zisimopoulou P, Rentzos M, et al. LRP4 antibodies in serum and CSF from amyotrophic lateral sclerosis patients. Ann Clin Transl Neurol 2014;1(2):80–7.
161. Cossins J, Belaya K, Zoltowska K, et al. The search for new antigenic targets in myasthenia gravis. Ann N Y Acad Sci 2012;1275:123–8.
162. Cortes-Vicente E, Gallardo E, Martinez MA, et al. Clinical characteristics of patients with double-seronegative myasthenia gravis and antibodies to cortactin. JAMA Neurol 2016;73(9):1099–104.

Treatment of Myasthenia Gravis

Constantine Farmakidis, MD, Mamatha Pasnoor, MD,
Mazen M. Dimachkie, MD*, Richard J. Barohn, MD

KEYWORDS

- Myasthenia gravis • Pyridostigmine • Prednisone • Thymectomy • Immunotherapy
- Complement inhibition • Intravenous immunoglobulin • Plasma exchange

KEY POINTS

- With advances in myasthenia gravis treatment, most patients have very good outcomes. The bedrock of MG treatment is immunotherapy, and symptomatic treatment with acetylcholinesterase inhibition.
- A recent international, rater-blinded, randomized trial provided strong evidence of improved clinical outcomes in acetylcholine receptor antibody positive nonthymomatous myasthenia gravis treated with thymectomy.
- In ocular disease, a randomized controlled trial found corticosteroids to be beneficial. Another recent trial failed to show a steroid-sparing effect in patients treated with methotrexate.
- A complement inhibitor, eculizumab was recently approved for the treatment of generalized myasthenia gravis. There are emerging therapies, including targeted monoclonal antibody agents that are currently under investigation.
- Patient recruitment continues to be a challenge in myasthenia gravis clinical trials.

Disclosure Statement: Drs C. Farmakidis and M. Pasnoor have nothing to disclose. Dr M.M. Dimachkie is on the speaker's bureau or is a consultant for Alnylam, Baxalta, Catalyst, CSL-Behring, Mallinckrodt, Novartis, NuFactor, and Terumo. He has also received grants from Alexion, Biomarin, Catalyst, CSL Behring, FDA/OPD, GSK, Grifols, MDA, NIH, Novartis, Orphazyme, Sanofi, and TMA. Dr R.J. Barohn is a consultant for NuFactor and is on the advisory board for Novartis. He has received an honorarium from Option Care and PlatformQ Health Education. He has received research grants from NIH, FDA/OOPD, NINDS, Novartis, Sanofi/Genzyme, Biomarin, IONIS, Teva, Cytokinetics, Eli Lilly, PCORI, ALSA, and PTC. This work was supported by a CTSA grant from NCATS awarded to the University of Kansas for Frontiers: University of Kansas Clinical and Translational Science Institute (# UL1TR002366) The contents are solely the responsibility of the authors and do not necessarily represent the official views of the NIH or NCATS.

Department of Neurology, University of Kansas Medical Center, 3901 Rainbow Boulevard, Mail Stop 2012, Kansas City, KS 66160, USA
* Corresponding author.
E-mail address: mdimachkie@kumc.edu

Neurol Clin 36 (2018) 311–337
https://doi.org/10.1016/j.ncl.2018.01.011
0733-8619/18/© 2018 Elsevier Inc. All rights reserved.

INTRODUCTION

Myasthenia gravis (MG) is the most common acquired disorder of neuromuscular transmission. It occurs due to the production of pathogenic autoantibodies that bind to components of the neuromuscular junction, the most common being the acetylcholinesterase receptor (AChR). The incidence is estimated at 0.3 to 2.8 per 100,000 and the worldwide prevalence at 700,000.[1] In 1934, cholinesterase inhibition was demonstrated as the first effective treatment for MG.[2] Until the last 20 years, most MG treatment was investigated through retrospective clinical studies. More recently, there have been a number of randomized controlled clinical trials (**Box 1**). The decades that various MG treatments were introduced is shown in **Box 2**. This development has been associated with dramatic improvements in survival and prognosis in MG.[3] The primary reasons for reduced mortality rates are the improvement in intensive respiratory care and the introduction of immunosuppressive treatments. Although the mortality rate was previously quite high, resulting in the name MG, the current mortality rate in MG is reported as 0.06 to 0.89 per million person-years.[4]

Box 1
Myasthenia gravis treatment: controlled randomized trials

1. Mount 1964 – Adrenocorticotrophic hormone versus placebo.
2. Howard 1976 – Alternate day prednisone versus placebo[a]
3. Tindall 1987 – Cyclosporine versus placebo/virgin patients[a,b]
4. Tindall 1993 – Cyclosporine versus placebo/immunosuppressed patients[a,b]
5. Gajdos 1997 – Plasma exchange versus intravenous immunoglobulin[b]
6. Lindberg 1998 – Pulse methylprednisone versus placebo[a,b]
7. Palace 1998 – Azathioprine/prednisone versus azathioprine/placebo[a,b]
8. Wolfe 2002 – Intravenous immunoglobulin versus placebo[a]
9. Meriggioli 2003 – Mycophenolate mofetil versus placebo[a]
10. Gajdos 2005 – Intravenous immunoglobulin – 2 doses[a,b]
11. Nagane 2005 – Tacrolimus versus placebo[b]
12. Sanders/MSG 2008 – Mycophenolate mofetil versus placebo[a]
13. Sanders/Aspreva 2008 – Mycophenolate mofetil versus placebo[a]
14. Zinman 2007 – Intravenous immunoglobulin versus placebo[a,b]
15. Soliven 2008 – Terbutaline versus placebo[a,b]
16. Barth 2011 – Intravenous immunoglobulin versus plasma exchange[b]
17. Heckmann 2011 - Methotrexate versus azathioprine[a,b]
18. Howard 2013 - Eculizumab versus placebo[b]
19. Benatar 2013 – Prednisone for ocular myasthenia[b]
20. Pasnoor/Barohn 2014: Methotrexate versus placebo[a]
21. Wolfe 2016 - Transsternal thymectomy in generalized myasthenia[b]
22. Howard 2016- Eculizumab versus placebo, Phase 3[a] (FDA approved 2017)

[a] Blinded.
[b] Positive trials.

| Box 2 |
| Treatments for myasthenia gravis and decade introduced |
| 1930s: physostigmine, neostigmine |
| 1940s: thymectomy |
| 1950s: mechanical ventilation, edrophonium chloride, pyridostigmine |
| 1960s: corticosteroids and plasma exchange |
| 1970s: azathioprine |
| 1980s: cyclosporine, cyclophosphamide |
| 1990s: intravenous immunoglobulin |
| 2000s: mycophenolate mofetil, tacrolimus |
| 2010s: rituximab, eculizumab |

The various treatments for MG and the approximate time lag to onset of action are outlined in **Table 1**.

In this review, we summarize information on most MG treatment modalities and offer recommendations for the management of generalized MG and MG crises.

SYMPTOMATIC TREATMENT
Anticholinesterase Inhibitors

Acetylcholinesterase inhibitors were discovered and introduced into medical practice during the 19th century.[5] In 1934, Walker hypothesized that physostigmine, an agent used as a partial antagonist to curare, may counteract the curare poisoning-like features of MG and described rapid onset and dramatic but temporary improvement in a 56-year-old woman with generalized MG.[2,6] She followed this with a brief and also positive report of prostigmine for generalized MG.[7] Prostigmine was the acetylcholinesterase inhibitor of the time from the mid-1930s to the mid-1950s, when pyridostigmine was introduced.[8–11] To our knowledge, branded Prostigmin is no longer available in the United States, but generic neostigmine is.

Pyridostigmine, a synthetic acetylcholinesterase inhibitor, inhibits the hydrolysis of the acetylcholine neurotransmitter in the synaptic cleft. This agent increases the number of interactions between the acetylcholine and the acetylcholine receptor in the neuromuscular junction. Pyridostigmine does not cross the blood–brain barrier, thereby limiting central nervous system toxicity, and may be mildly effective in ocular and generalized MG.

A typical starting dose is 60 mg every 6 hours during daytime hours (see **Table 1**). Dosage may be titrated up to 60 to 120 mg every 3 hours aiming to minimize symptoms, but at these higher doses side effects are more likely to occur. Clinical effect onset is 15 to 30 minutes and its duration is about 3 to 4 hours. For patients who awaken at night or in the morning with impairing weakness, a 180-mg extended release formulation of pyridostigmine may be taken before sleep. However, owing to uneven absorption and unpredictable effect, the use of this medication has been limited.

Gastrointestinal side effects such as abdominal cramping, loose stools, and flatulence are most common. Increased perspiration and muscle twitches and cramps are other side effects. Acetylcholinesterase inhibitors are relatively contraindicated in myasthenic crisis because they can increase secretions and complicate airway management. At very high doses, acetylcholinesterase inhibitors can precipitate a paradoxic increase in weakness with respiratory insufficiency, a condition recognized

Table 1
Summary and treatment recommendations for myasthenia gravis

Therapy	Starting Dose	Maintenance Dose	Onset of Action	Adverse Events	Monitoring	Comment
First-line therapies						
Pyridostigmine	60 mg every 6 h while awake	60–120 mg every 3–8 h while awake	15–30 min	Loose stools, n/v, diarrhea	None	Patients can learn over time to adjust dosage; with current dosing, cholinergic crisis is rare
Prednisone	Rapid induction regimen: 60–100 mg/d for 2–4 wk; slow titration regimen: 10 mg/d, increase by 10 mg every 5–7 d up to 60–100 mg	60–100 mg/d, followed by a slow alternate day taper	2–4 wk	HTN, hyperglycemia, fluid retention, weight gain, bone density loss, neuropsychiatric	Weight, BP, glucose, potassium, bone density monitoring	With high doses, watch for early worsening. Seen in as many as half of patients; single morning dose; minimize long-term exposure
Thymectomy	—	—	6–12 mo	—	—	See text
Second-line therapies						
Azathioprine	50 mg, single morning dose	Increase by 50 mg every 2–4 wk; goal dose 2–3 mg/kg/d	12–18 mo	Flu-like illness, n/v, hepatotoxicity; leukopenia	CBC, LFTs monthly. Weekly only for first month	Major drug interaction with allopurinol; uncertain degree of fetal risk in pregnancy
Cyclosporine	100 mg twice daily	Goal dose 3–6 mg/kg/d, divided in 2 daily doses	1–3 mo	Nephrotoxicity, HTN, infection, hepatotoxicity, hirsutism, tremor, gum hyperplasia, neoplasia	BP, monthly cyclosporine trough level <300 ng/mL, BUN/Cr, LFTs, CBC	Different preparations/ brands are not bioequivalent and should not be mixed; trough level goal 100–150 ng/mL; watch for medication interactions

Intravenous Immunoglobulin	2 g/kg divided over 2–5 d	0.4–1 g/kg every 4 wk; try to decrease frequency over time	1–2 wk	Headache, urticaria, nephrotoxic, thrombotic events	BUN/Cr	Avoid in patients with recent thrombotic event; can pretreat with APAP 1000 mg PO for headache prophylaxis; with diphenhydramine 25 mg PO for urticaria prophylaxis
Third-line therapies						
Methotrexate	10 mg/wk	Increase by 2.5 mg every 2 wk, up to 20 mg/wk	—	Hepatotoxicity, pulmonary fibrosis, infection, neoplasia	Monthly LFT, CBC	Consider liver biopsy at 2 g cumulative dose
Mycophenolate mofetil	500 mg twice daily	1000–1500 mg twice daily	2–12 mo	Diarrhea, nausea, emesis, leukopenia	Monthly CBC, twice for first month	Risk of fetal harm including teratogenicity
Plasmapheresis	One plasma volume exchanged per procedure; 5 procedures every other day	—	~2 exchanges	Hypotension, hypocalcemia, fever, urticaria, infection, pneumothorax, PE	Blood pressure, calcium	Venous access preferable when available; Not infrequent but mild complications; In centers with significant experience discontinuation rates low
Fourth-line therapies						
Rituximab	375 mg/mm² given weekly for 4 wk; 750 mg/mm² given twice and 2 wk apart	Cycle may be repeated at 6 mo as needed	1–3 mo	Infusion-related headache, nausea, chills, hypotension; anemia, leukopenia, thrombocytopenia	Frequent CBC in first month; then monthly	Can pretreat with APAP 1000 mg PO for headache prophylaxis; with diphenhydramine 25 mg PO for pruritus prophylaxis

(continued on next page)

Table 1
(continued)

Fifth-line therapies

Therapy	Starting Dose	Maintenance Dose	Onset of Action	Adverse Events	Monitoring	Comment
Eculizumab	900 mg/wk for 4 wk; 1200 mg for the fifth week; and 1200 mg every 2 wk thereafter	1200 mg every 2 wk	2–4 wk	Mild infusion-related adverse events; life-threatening and fatal meningococcal infections have occurred	Likely CBC and complete metabolic profile	Must administer meningococcal vaccination before starting therapy. May pretreat with APAP 1000 mg PO and diphenhydramine 25 mg PO for headache and pruritus prophylaxis
Cyclophosphamide	0.5–1 g/m² IV induction dose	0.5–1 g/m² IV monthly maintenance dose for 6 mo; adjust dose based on trough neutrophil count	6–12 mo	Bone marrow suppression, infertility, hemorrhagic cystitis, alopecia, infections, neoplasia, teratogenicity, nausea	Daily to weekly CBC with attention to trough absolute neutrophil count; urinalysis	Must hydrate IV; must administer antiemetics and consider bladder prophylaxis for hemorrhagic cystitis

Abbreviations: APAP, acetaminophen; BP, blood pressure; BUN, blood urea nitrogen; CBC, complete blood count; Cr, creatinine; HTN, hypertension; IV, intravenous; LFT, liver function tests; n/v, nausea, vomiting; PE, pulmonary embolus.

as a cholinergic crisis. However, in the current era of effective immunotherapy, these extremely high doses are not used, and the cholinergic crisis has become more of a theoretic concern. Pyridostigmine can be used long term, and its effectiveness generally does not diminish over time. For the management of intrusive muscarinic side effects, options include oral glycopyrrolate 1 mg, hyoscyamine 0.125 mg, or loperamide 2 mg. Either drug can be taken concurrently with pyridostigmine doses, up to 3 times a day.

Data exist to guide the use of acetylcholinesterase inhibitors in different MG patient subgroups. Patients with muscle-specific kinase (MuSK) autoantibody-positive disease have lower response rates than patients with the AChR autoantibody.[12,13] Juvenile patients with MG may have a particularly robust acetylcholinesterase inhibitor response.[14] Patients with ocular MG, and particularly those with diplopia, frequently seem to not fully respond to acetylcholinesterase inhibitors, although ptosis seems to be more responsive than ocular paresis.[15,16] The apparent limited response in patients with diplopia may be because, unless the ocular motility is completely restored, some degree of diplopia will persist.

CORTICOSTEROIDS

Corticosteroid treatment was the first widely used immunosuppressive therapy introduced in MG. The first reports of a beneficial response in MG involved high-dose prednisone (100 mg/d or every other day).[17,18] Early clinical studies showed prednisone's dramatic impact on myasthenic patients, with 80% or more showing either medical remission or marked improvement.[19] Although evidence from randomized controlled clinical trials remains limited and side effects pose significant challenges in clinical use, corticosteroids are considered the most effective oral immunosuppressive agent and are widely recommended as a first-line agent for use in patients with MG.[20–23] Although corticosteroids are known to have a broad inhibitory effect on immune response via the reduction of endothelial adhesion of leukocytes and a decrease in inflammatory cytokine production, the exact mechanism of action in MG remains unknown. Studies of the effect of corticosteroids therapy on acetylcholine receptor antibody titers have shown conflicting results with both decreased and unchanged antibody titers. This finding possibly implies an effect on cell-mediated immunity for corticosteroids in MG.

The clinical response to corticosteroids can start within days, and most patients experience initial benefits within the first 2 weeks.[19] Patients attain maximal improvement on corticosteroids in the first 6 months, although some may take as long as 2 years or more.[19] There are 2 prevalent approaches to oral corticosteroids administration: a high-dose, rapid treatment induction regimen, and a low-dose and slow titration regimen (see **Table 1**). The slow titration regimen is designed to reduce the risk of initial worsening seen in as many as one-half the patients started on corticosteroids, but more commonly in the patient subset with severe MG or marked bulbar manifestations. The high-dose regimen consists of prednisone 1.0 to 1.5 mg/kg/d (but usually not >100 mg/d) for 2 to 4 weeks. After this period, a decision is made to immediately switch to every other day or to continue daily high-dose therapy. Switching immediately to alternate day high-dose corticosteroids may be used for patients who are Myasthenia Gravis Foundation of America (MGFA) grade 2 (mild). However, higher grade patients with MG usually require daily corticosteroid dosing for extended periods. Whether the patient is switched to a higher daily dosing at 2 to 4 weeks or left on high-dose daily therapy, the patient is usually kept on that dose (eg, 100 mg every other day or 50 mg/d) for another

4 to 8 weeks, at which time improvement should be noted and a slow taper by 5 to 10 mg a month can be initiated.

A low-dose and slow titration regimen is suited for patients with milder disability, including ocular MG or in mild to moderate MG. In the low-dose approach, 10 mg/d is administered, and the prednisone is increased by 10 mg every 5 to 7 days to a peak dose of 1.0 to 1.5 mg/kg/d (up to 60–100 mg).[24] A third and more recent approach is based on the mycophenolate mofetil study,[25] and it places patients on a fixed dose of prednisone 20 mg immediately, monitoring that dose, unless there is no response, and then the dose should be increased. We have been using the 20 mg/d and stay approach since the mycophenolate mofetil study, and have found that it is often successful, as in the mycophenolate study. We believe that a comparative effectiveness study of different prednisone dosing approaches in MG is warranted.

Daily prednisone use is also the rule for patients in myasthenic crisis and for those with worsening symptoms but who are not yet in crisis. A switch to alternate day prednisone can be made months later, when the patient has begun to improve significantly. A daily long-term steroid regimen may be indicated in patients with diabetes and hypertension to avoid wide swings in serum glucose and blood pressure, respectively.

In ocular MG, the use of corticosteroids has been the subject of debate, weighing the considerable functional impairment from diplopia and ptosis against the risk of significant systemic toxicity from chronic corticosteroid use.[26] A recent small randomized, double-blind trial of prednisone 10 mg every other day titrated up to 40 mg/d over 16 weeks versus placebo in patients with ocular MG showed that 100% of the placebo group patients (n = 5) failed to improve, whereas only 17% of the prednisone group (n = 6) failed to improve (P = .02).[20] The strength of this evidence is limited by a small sample size, but this study indicates that prednisone can be an effective treatment for ocular MG and should be considered in patients that fail acetylcholinesterase inhibitors. This small but dramatically positive study is probably the best randomized controlled trial of prednisone in MG.

Several retrospective studies have provided evidence that immunotherapy (including treatment with corticosteroids) may reduce the risk of developing generalized MG in patients with ocular MG.[27,28] In the largest of these studies, after 2 years of follow-up, 36% of patients not treated on prednisone progressed to generalized MG versus only 7% of patients treated with prednisone.[27] In another retrospective study, pyridostigmine was used without prednisone in 59 of 97 patients with ocular MG with 12 developing generalized MG, whereas none of the 38 prednisone-treated cases developed generalized MG.[16]

The systemic side effects of long-term corticosteroid therapy are numerous and can be highly impactful. They include weight gain, diabetes, hypertension, eye disease (cataract and glaucoma), accelerated bone demineralization, and neuropsychiatric disturbances. Potential complications should be discussed before the initiation of treatment, and prevention and monitoring plans should be established in collaboration with the patient's primary care physician. We recommend placing a tuberculin skin test or obtaining a QuantiFERON-TB Gold test to identify patients previously exposed to tuberculosis before starting corticosteroids therapy. Prophylactic therapy is indicated in those who test positive for prior exposure. Patients should be counseled about a low carbohydrate, low calorie, and low salt diet. If the patient is hospitalized, this can be done by the dietician. However, dieticians are often not available in the outpatient setting and, therefore, it is up to the neurologist to provide some dietary guidance. The advice of "no junk food/no salt when food gets to the table" is a good starting point, and should be reinforced on follow-up visits. A dual energy x-ray absorptiometry scan and an ophthalmologic examination should be obtained at baseline and repeated annually. Calcium (500 mg 2 to 3 times daily) and vitamin D (400 IU/d) supplements should be taken to reduce the risk of pathologic fractures. Patients should also remain up to date on all vaccinations, including the flu and pneumococcal vaccines, but no live or live attenuated vaccines should be used by patients on immunotherapy.[29]

OTHER IMMUNOSUPPRESSANTS
Azathioprine

Azathioprine is a purine synthesis cytotoxic antimetabolite that inhibits DNA and RNA synthesis, cellular replication, and lymphocyte function. The use of azathioprine for MG therapy was pioneered in Europe in the 1970s, and azathioprine has become the most widely accepted steroid-sparing immunosuppressant used for MG.[22,30] In comparison with other steroid-sparing options, azathioprine has more favorable tolerability, although a major challenge in its clinical use is the estimated 6- to 18-month latency between treatment initiation and therapeutic onset.[31,32]

A number of earlier retrospective studies have suggested response rates to azathioprine ranging from 70% to 91%.[30,33] There has been 1 randomized, double-blind clinical trial of oral prednisolone plus azathioprine 2.5 mg/kg/d versus oral prednisolone and placebo.[32] Enrollment was slow, took several years to complete it. Patients were observed over 3 years and the corticosteroid dose was adjusted up or down to the lowest dose necessary to maintain pharmacologic remission. Thirty-four patients were enrolled, but the dropout rate was high. At 12 months, there was no significant difference in the prednisolone dose between both groups (N = 24; placebo 15 cases and azathioprine 9), but there was a trend for a lower prednisolone dose in the azathioprine group. At 18 months, there was a statistically significant difference in the prednisolone dose between the 2 groups. At 3 years, most patients in the prednisolone plus azathioprine group (n = 8) had been successfully tapered off steroids. Weight gain was also less in the prednisolone plus azathioprine group compared with the prednisolone and placebo group, at 2 kg/y and 5.8 kg/y, respectively. Conversely, in the prednisolone and placebo groups, patients were more likely to fail to remit and to relapse even with the flaws noted. This is an important positive study in the MG field and supports the use of azathioprine. However, azathioprine may not improve an MG patient in the first year of treatment and is used for long-term management to get patients on lower corticosteroids doses or off corticosteroids altogether.

Azathioprine has been used in patients with generalized MG on corticosteroids who are still symptomatic; in patients with relative contraindications to corticosteroids treatment such as hypertension, diabetes, and osteoporosis; and in those who experience severe side effects to corticosteroids. Azathioprine has also been used in patients with ocular MG requiring but not tolerating corticosteroid therapy.[34]

The starting dose for azathioprine is 50 mg/d (see **Table 1**). Dosing can be increased in 50-mg increments every 2 to 4 weeks to a goal dose of 2 to 3 mg/kg/d. Blood counts and liver function should be tested at baseline, and then monthly. An important monitoring parameter of bone marrow suppression is the white blood count and leukopenia.[35] Others include liver function test evaluation (alanine aminotransferase, aspartate aminotransferase). We monitor a complete blood count and a complete metabolic panel. If the white blood cell count decreases to less than 4000 mm^3, we decrease the azathioprine dose, and if it decreases to less than 3000 per mm^3, we stop the drug. We also monitor the absolute neutrophil count to make sure it is not affected, but expect some lymphopenia in the range of 500 to

1000 per mm³. If the aspartate aminotransferase or alanine aminotransferase levels elevate, we stop the drug. When the liver enzymes return to normal the patient can be rechallenged and occasionally this measure can be effective without enzyme elevations.

In rheumatic diseases and in posttransplant care, azathioprine has been linked to a higher risk of developing a malignancy, although a parallel phenomenon has not been described in patients with MG.[36] Although evidence from the transplant literature indicates that the risk for adverse outcomes from azathioprine use in pregnancy is very low, we do not use azathioprine in pregnancy.

Of the patients placed on azathioprine, 10% to 20% have an idiosyncratic drug reaction presenting as a flulike syndrome with fever, malaise, and loss of appetite.[29] This phenomenon occurs in the first 1 to 2 weeks after starting the drug. If it occurs, azathioprine should be stopped immediately, and the symptoms will lessen in a day or two. If azathioprine is restarted, these side effects almost always recur.

It has been suggested that before initiation of azathioprine, thiopurine methyltransferase phenotype or genotype be tested as an inherited enzyme deficiency predicts an increased risk for leukopenia. A systematic review of 55 studies found that, although diminished TMPT activity is associated with myelotoxicity, there is insufficient evidence to support screening patients for thiopurine methyltransferase deficiency.[37] In practice, we monitor blood cell counts closely instead.

Mycophenolate Mofetil

Similar to other newer immunosuppressants, mycophenolate mofetil was introduced in neuromuscular diseases after initial experience as an antirejection drug in transplant medicine.[38] Mycophenolate mofetil is a potent monophosphate dehydrogenase inhibitor. It inhibits guanosine nucleotide synthesis that is essential for B and T lymphocytes. Initial interest was spurred in MG after the report of a patient with treatment-refractory early-onset myasthenia who had a rapid response to mycophenolate mofetil.[39] Several retrospective studies suggested a favorable tolerability profile, the potential for a prednisone-sparing effect, and robust rates of disease control around 70%.[40,41] In addition, in comparison with azathioprine, a more rapid initial clinical response time (11 weeks) was suggested.

However, both of 2 large multicenter, randomized, double-blinded, placebo-controlled trials failed to show that mycophenolate mofetil in addition to prednisone was more effective in controlling MG. In 1 study, 80 patients with mild to moderate generalized AChR antibody–positive MG were randomized to 20 mg/d of prednisone plus 2.5 g/d mycophenolate mofetil versus 20 mg/d prednisone and placebo and followed over 12 weeks.[25] The primary outcome was change in the Quantitative Myasthenia Gravis (QMG) score, which was similarly decreased in both groups, indicating there was no advantage detected in the mycophenolate mofetil group. Both groups improved which implies a significant effect of prednisone 20 mg/d. In the international phase III mycophenolate mofetil study, 176 AChR antibody–positive patients with mild to moderate MG who were already taking corticosteroids were randomized to mycophenolate mofetil 2 g/d versus placebo.[42] At the conclusion of 36 weeks (9 months), the primary endpoint measured—which was a composite of a favorable MGFA postintervention status and prednisone and pyridostigmine doses below certain preset ceiling levels—did not show the mycophenolate mofetil group outperforming the placebo group.

The discordance between the retrospective and randomized trial data of mycophenolate mofetil has several potential explanations. The most favored is that the therapeutic potency of 20 mg of prednisone may have been underestimated and thus overwhelmed the therapeutic effect of mycophenolate mofetil. It is also possible that clinical trial periods were not long enough to capture the onset of the effect of mycophenolate mofetil, or that the disease population studied was too mildly affected to require both prednisone and mycophenolate mofetil for treatment. Since the publication of these negative randomized, controlled trials, another retrospective study provided evidence of benefit for mycophenolate mofetil, although the strength of the evidence is limited by its retrospective design.[43] Despite 2 negative studies, mycophenolate mofetil is listed as part of the international consensus guidance for MG management.[22] In our practice, although we still use mycophenolate mofetil for some patients with MG, we do not use it quite as often since the publication of these 2 randomized controlled trials. The most common regimens used are 1000 to 1500 mg twice daily (see **Table 1**). The main side effects are diarrhea, nausea, infections, and leukopenia. Blood counts should be monitored closely at the initiation of treatment and thereafter monthly, and we use the same guidelines for dosing adjustment outlined for azathioprine. Mycophenolate mofetil is contraindicated in pregnancy owing to teratogenic potential and a higher risk of miscarriage in the first 3 months.[44] Concerns exist regarding a potential increase in the risk of lymphoproliferative disease based on isolated case reports.[45,46]

Cyclosporine

Cyclosporine, an agent first used to suppress allograft rejection, interferes with calcineurin signaling, suppresses cytokine secretion including interleukin-2 and interferon-γ, and interferes with T-helper cell activation. Cyclosporine was the first immunosuppressant medication shown to be effective in the treatment of generalized MG in 2 small double-blind, randomized, controlled trials.[47,48]

In the first randomized trial, newly diagnosed, thymectomy- and immunosuppression-naïve generalized patients with MG were treated with cyclosporine 6 mg/kg/d versus placebo. The cyclosporine level was monitored, and the dose adjusted to maintain trough levels between 400 and 600 ng/mL and creatinine at 2.0 mg/dL or less. At 6 months, the cyclosporine group had a lower QMG score compared with the placebo group, and that persisted and remained statistically significant at 12 months.[47] In a second randomized, controlled trial of cyclosporine, a group of steroid-dependent patients ($\geq$30 mg of prednisone every other day) with or without a thymectomy, and with varying degrees of prior immunosuppressive therapy was treated with 5 mg/kg/d of cyclosporine versus placebo with the cyclosporine dose adjusted to maintain trough levels between 300 and 500 ng/mL and creatinine of 2.0 mg/dL or less.[48] At the conclusion of the study at 6 months, the cyclosporine group had a lower QMG score, had a greater reduction of AChR antibody levels, and was on a lower prednisone dose, although this lower dose was not statistically significant. In an 18-month, open-label extension of the study, the steroid-sparing effect of cyclosporine seemed to increase.

Acute and more indolently progressive renal toxicity and hypertension are major factors limiting the tolerability of cyclosporine. Serum creatinine levels in a case series increased by a mean of 48% in more than one-quarter of treated patients and the cumulative side effects led to the discontinuation of treatment in 35% of patients over a 2-year period.[48,49] There is also evidence that cyclosporine is associated with increased dermatologic and other malignancy risk.[49] In addition to increased skin surveillance and measures to limit sun exposure, the neoplasia risk of cyclosporine should be reviewed individually before initiating treatment. Other limiting side effects are hirsutism, tremor, gum hyperplasia, paresthesias, headaches, and hepatotoxicity.

The starting dose of cyclosporine is usually 3 mg/kg/d (see **Table 1**) and it comes in 100 mg capsules. Thus, a 70-kg person generally takes 200 mg split in 2 doses. Similar to corticosteroids, the goal is to reduce cyclosporine to the lowest dose that maintains treatment effect. Trough levels should be monitored (keep at <300 ng/mL) as well as serum creatinine, blood urea nitrogen, and liver function tests. Different cyclosporine preparations should not be mixed owing to differing pharmacokinetics, and the patient' medication lists should be screened before the initiation of this drug because a number of medications interact with cyclosporine and destabilize serum drug levels.

Tacrolimus, a similar agent to cyclosporine, also seems to have a beneficial effect in MG, as shown in a small randomized pilot study.[50] In another study, a cohort of 13 children aged 7 to 13 years were treated for 1 year with tacrolimus 1 to 2 mg/d for MG poorly responsive to prednisone.[51] The prednisone dose was significantly decreased, with improvement in MG symptoms as assessed by the QMG, MG Manual Muscle Testing, and MG Activities of Daily Living and reduction of anti-AChR antibody titers. Most patients were able to completely discontinue prednisone.

Methotrexate

Methotrexate is a folate antimetabolite that inhibits dihydrofolate reductase. When given in high doses as part of a cancer chemotherapy regimen, methotrexate has a distinct cytotoxic effect; at lower doses, methotrexate induces an immunomodulatory effect, the mechanism of which is not fully understood.[52] A small randomized, single-blinded study of methotrexate in MG compared methotrexate 17.5 mg/wk with daily prednisone as compared with azathioprine at 2.5 to 3.0 mg/kg/d with daily prednisone.[53] At 2 years there was a substantial and comparable decrease in the average daily prednisone dose and the QMG scores in both groups. These data suggested a similar efficacy between azathioprine and methotrexate over a 2-year period, although with a cost advantage for methotrexate. A randomized, double-blind, placebo-controlled trial of methotrexate 20 mg/wk by mouth versus placebo in prednisone-dependent patients with MG was designed to more definitively determine if methotrexate is effective as a corticosteroid-sparing agent.[54] The results using the predetermined intention-to-treat multiple imputation analysis showed no difference in the prednisone area under the curve between methotrexate and placebo over a 12-month observation period. Primary analysis of the secondary outcomes (QMG, MG Activities of Daily Living, etc) similarly showed no difference between the 2 groups. However, there were more patients in the placebo group that dropped out owing to worsening MG. In addition, a post hoc analysis using other intention-to-treat methods (last-dose-carried forward, worst/highest dose carried forward) showed methotrexate patients had significantly lower QMG, MG Activities of Daily Living and MG Composite scores (**Table 2**).

As in the mycophenolate trials, this study raised the question of whether the drug is ineffective, or whether the trial's sensitivity was limited by concurrent corticosteroids treatment, insufficiently long follow-up, a small study sample, or incorrectly chosen intention-to-treat design.

As a third-line agent, methotrexate is started at 10 mg/wk and titrated to 20 mg/wk over 2 months (see **Table 1**). We also give folic acid 1 mg/d to prevent stomatitis and monitor for bone marrow suppression and liver toxicity. Methotrexate is strictly contraindicated in women who may become pregnant and should be used cautiously in patients with lung pathology because it is rarely associated with pulmonary fibrosis.

Table 2
Methotrexate study sensitivity analysis

Outcome Measures	Multiple Imputation MTX Versus Placebo, Mean/Median (SE)[a]	P Value[b]	Last Dose/Score Carried Forward MTX Versus Placebo, Mean/Median (SE)[a]	P Value[b]	Highest Dose/Worst Value Carried Forward for Worsening Cases MTX Versus Placebo Mean/Median (SE)[a]	P Value[b]
Primary outcome						
Median 9-mo prednisone AUDTC, mg	2996.6 (727.1) vs 3484.7 (645.8)	.26	3330.0 (718.8) vs 3679.0 (748.0)	.27	3330.0 (718.8) vs 3679.0 (591.1)	.20
Median prednisone daily dose, mg/d	11.9 (2.9) vs 13.8 (2.6)	.26	13.2 (2.9) vs 14.6 (3.0)	.27	13.2 (2.9) vs 14.6 (2.3)	.20
Secondary outcomes						
Mean 12-mo QMG change	−1.4 (0.7) vs 0.3 (1.0)	.29	−1.6 (0.7) vs 1.4 (0.9)	.01	−1.6 (0.7) vs 1.5 (0.9)	.01
Mean 12-mo MMT change	−5.5 (0.9) vs −3.3 (1.6)	.28	−5.7 (0.9) vs −3.0 (1.6)	.16	−5.7 (0.9) vs −2.6 (1.6)	.11
Median 12-mo MG-QOL change	−4.6 (4.5) vs −3.7 (4.8)	.82	−3.0 (2.0) vs −2.0 (1.5)	.18	−3.0 (1.9) vs −1(1.4)	.15
Mean 12-mo MG-ADL change	−1.2 (0.5) vs −0.3 (0.6)	.21	−1.2 (0.5) vs 0.48 (0.5)	.02	−1.2 (0.5) vs 0.5 (0.5)	.02
Mean 12-mo MGC change	−4.6 (0.9) vs −1.3 (1.1)	.09	−4.7(0.9) vs −1.1 (1.1)	.02	−4.7 (0.9) vs −0.9 (1.1)	.01

Abbreviations: AUDTC, area under the dose-time curve; MG-ADL, Myasthenia Gravis Activities of Daily Living Scale; MGC, Myasthenia Gravis Composite score; MG-QOL, Myasthenia Gravis Quality of Life Scale; MMT, manual muscle testing; MTX, methotrexate; QMG, Quantitative Myasthenia Gravis score; SE, standard error.

[a] Mean (SE) were used as summary statistics if normality assumption was satisfied; otherwise, median (SE) were used as summary statistics (prednisone 9-mo AUDTC, prednisone daily dose, and MG-QOL). The SEs for medians were estimated by bootstrapping.

[b] The 2-sample *t* test was used if normality assumption was satisfied; otherwise, the Wilcoxon rank-sum test was used. For the primary outcome, a significance level of .05 was used, and for the secondary outcomes, .01 was used to adjust for multiple comparisons.

Data from Dimachkie MM. Idiopathic inflammatory myopathies. J Neuroimmunol 2011;231(1–2):32–42 and Barohn RJ, Dimachkie MM. Tratamientos inmunomoduladores. In: Mazia C, ed. Miastenia Gravis Y Problemas Relacionados. Buenos Aires: Inter-Médica; 2017:273–89.

Cyclophosphamide

Cyclophosphamide is an alkylating agent that modifies the guanine base of DNA, conferring cytotoxic properties. This action in turn suppresses bone marrow cell replication and B- and T-cell immune function. A case series and a small, randomized double-blind clinical trial have provided evidence that cyclophosphamide both improves weakness and also has steroid-sparing effect in MG.[55,56]

In a randomized, controlled trial of 500 mg/m^2 monthly intravenous cyclophosphamide pulses, those in the cyclophosphamide arm had a significantly improved QMG score at month 12 and a lower steroid dose at months 6 and 12.[56] Drachman and associates[57] described long-lasting improvement in 3 patients with refractory disease treated with "rebooting of the immune system" through intravenous cyclophosphamide 50 mg/kg for 4 days, followed by rescue with granulocyte colony stimulating factor. The associated toxicity is, however, considerable with alopecia reported in 75%, leukopenia in 35%, and nausea and vomiting in 25% of patients and the increased risk of hemorrhagic cystitis.[55] Cyclophosphamide remains an option for severe and refractory MG. However, owing to a poor tolerability profile and the advent of alternative immunotherapy, cyclophosphamide is used only rarely for MG.

Rituximab

Rituximab is a genetically engineered chimeric mouse–human monoclonal antibody directed against CD20, a transmembrane protein selectively found on the surface of normal and malignant B-lymphocytes.[58] Rituximab decreases the number of circulating CD20$^+$ B cells and is also thought to suppress antibody production and humoral immunity. A case of a treatment-resistant MG patient with an apparent response to rituximab provided initial evidence that rituximab may have a role in MG treatment.[59]

Rituximab therapy in MG is supported by demonstrable defects in B-cell tolerance checkpoints in MG.[60] These investigators identified defects in B cells, some of which were large-scale abnormalities in B-cell antibody repertoires that were unique to either AChR MG or MuSK MG. These findings suggest that the repertoires reflect the distinct properties of these 2 MG subtypes and that perhaps treatment response may be different in AChR MG from MuSK MG. Nonetheless, retrospective reports have provided additional evidence for a role for rituximab in MG.[61] In patients with MuSK MG, a particular subgroup otherwise known to be less responsive to standard therapies, retrospective data suggest that rituximab may have a more robust and persistent treatment effect.[62,63]

A recent systematic review of available retrospective rituximab studies found that the Modified MFGA postintervention scale of minimal manifestation status or better was attained in 72% of MuSK patients, 30% of AChR antibody patients, and 44% in both groups combined.[58] The strongest predictors for a clinical response were a positive MuSK antibody status, less severe disease, and younger age at the time of treatment.

The optimal rituximab dosing for MG is not established. A commonly used induction regimen is 375 mg/m^2 infusions given weekly for 4 weeks (see **Table 1**).[58,64] Another method that we often use is to administer 1 g and in 2 weeks administer another 1-g dose. Patients can be redosed every 4 to 6 months, but for how long is not known. Also unknown is the benefit of measuring B-cell counts (CD20) before the next dose is given. We do not do this routinely. Progressive multifocal encephalopathy (PML) is a feared complication of rituximab therapy that occurs after reactivation of the JC virus. To date, only 1 patient has been reported with PML in the setting of rituximab therapy for MG, and notably in the setting of prior longstanding use of other immunosuppressants.[65] A recent study reported a large series of PML cases in the setting of rituximab and natalizumab therapy, mostly for lymphoproliferative and rheumatic diseases.[66] This study suggested that older age and male sex are risk factors for developing PML.

A multicenter randomized, controlled trial of rituximab in generalized MG has completed recruitment.[67] The primary outcome measure investigated is the percent of patients achieving a 75% or greater reduction in the mean daily steroid dose recorded over the last month of a 12-month follow-up period and frequency of study-related adverse events.

RAPID-ACTING IMMUNOTHERAPIES
Plasma Exchange

Plasma exchange (PLEX) has garnered wide acceptance as an effective treatment in patients with MG since initial reports of its use in the late 1970s.[68,69] Unfortunately, no adequate randomized, controlled trial has been performed to evaluate whether PLEX improves long- or short-term outcomes in MG; however, there is indirect evidence for benefit. While early in the use of plasmapheresis for neuromuscular disease, a randomized Guillain-Barré Syndrome study was done in North America comparing plasmapheresis with care without plasmapheresis.[70] Such a study was never done in MG. This was highlighted in the American Academy of Neurology Therapeutic and Technology Awareness Subcommittee, which gave PLEX in MG crisis a level U (unknown whether it is effective or not) recommendation based on class III evidence.[71] Several randomized studies comparing the efficacy of PLEX with intravenous immunoglobulin (IVIG) showed that IVIG and PLEX had comparable therapeutic in patients with moderate to severe disease, and a few years earlier IVIG had been shown to be independently superior to placebo in MG.[72–74] Indications for a short-term course of PLEX are crises (MG grade 5, on mechanical ventilation), impending crisis in patients with severe MG (grade 4/4B) with dysphagia, respiratory dysfunction, or generalized weakness and when a patient with mild (2/2B) or moderate (3/3B) MG is worsening or not responding to other immunosuppressant therapies. An additional indication is prethymectomy in symptomatic patients to treat respiratory and bulbar weakness before surgery. In patients with highly refractory MG, chronic PLEX can be useful in long-term disease control, although no standard chronic treatment protocols have been evaluated systematically.

Venous access can be peripheral or central, although when adequate peripheral venous access is available it is preferable owing to the lower risks of peripheral vein cannulation. One standardized regimen used in clinical studies consists of 5 PLEX procedures where 1 plasma volume is exchanged per procedure and treatments occur every other day (see **Table 1**).[75] The replacement fluid used for plasma is 5% albumin with added calcium gluconate to prevent hypocalcemia and its clinical sequelae, known as the citrate effect. For patients who require central venous access, PLEX treatments may also be performed daily over 5 days to reduce the risk of a catheter-related infection.[75]

PLEX's mechanism of action is through the removal of plasma-soluble factors, including pathogenic autoantibodies and cytokines.[76] Clinical improvement typically starts by the third treatment. The rapid onset of treatment effect suggests PLEX may be a preferred intervention when a patient is rapidly worsening. The treatment effect lasts in the order of weeks and provides a window for intensifying immunosuppressive therapy. In a controlled trial of PLEX in patients with MG, at day 14 after a full course of PLEX, 65% of patients improved.[73]

Recently, additional considerations in the use of PLEX have emerged. A cross-sectional analysis of patients with MG in a nationwide inpatient database from the

United States treated with PLEX suggested that a greater than 2-day delay after admission in PLEX administration was associated with higher mortality and complication rates.[77] Furthermore a single-center, retrospective analysis of a 33-year experience with PLEX and IVIG in juvenile MG, suggested that unlike in adult-onset MG where IVIG and PLEX are thought to be comparable, in juvenile MG, response to PLEX is more consistent.[78]

Traditionally, PLEX has been viewed as difficult to prescribe, complicated to deliver, and limited by central catheter-related complications such as infection, pneumothorax, and thromboembolism, in addition to milder side effects such as fever, urticaria, hypocalcemia, and hypotension. Prospective data from 1727 successive PLEX treatments in 174 patients (13% with MG), however, showed that complications, although not infrequent, are minor and with very few treatment discontinuations or transitions to a higher level of care.[79] Similarly, a subanalysis of the PLEX arm in a single-center prospective PLEX and IVIG comparison study indicated that PLEX has the potential for very good tolerability when delivered in a center with significant expertise.[75] Specifically, 90% of patients with moderate to severe MG received PLEX as outpatients, 83% of patients completed PLEX via peripheral venous access, and adverse reactions were generally mild. In patients who require long-term PLEX and have difficult peripheral access, we have inserted arteriovenous fistulas in the arms with some success (**Fig. 1**).[80]

INTRAVENOUS IMMUNOGLOBULINS

Early uncontrolled studies suggested that IVIG is a safe and effective adjunctive treatment for MG.[81–83] A first randomized trial of IVIG in MG was cut short owing to logistical reasons (nationwide shortage of IVIG) and was inconclusive.[84] After demonstrating that PLEX and IVIG are equivalent therapies in MG acute exacerbation,[85] Gajdos and colleagues[86] reported in 2005 no superiority of IVIG 2 g/kg over 1 g/kg in treating acute MG exacerbation. A second randomized, double-blind, placebo-controlled trial compared the effect of 2 g/kg of IVIG over 2 days with an equivalent volume of placebo infusion in patients with MG with worsening weakness. The study, which was reported in 2007, found meaningful clinical improvement at 14 days via the QMG score in the IVIG group, although the magnitude of the improvement was surprisingly small. The potential for IVIG benefit effect may have been underreported, however, because many patients with milder disease were included in the study cohort. A subgroup analysis underscored this possibility, showing that only patients with moderate to severe disease had a significant treatment effect.[74] Nevertheless, to date this is the only positive randomized, controlled trial comparing IVIG with

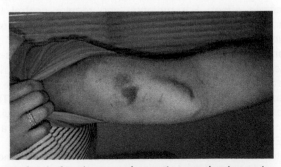

Fig. 1. Arteriovenous fistula for plasma exchange in myasthenia gravis.

placebo for MG. Currently, trials are underway by the pharmaceutical industry that, if positive, could lead to labeling indication from the US Food and Drug Administration of IVIG for MG.

IVIG has a complex immunomodulatory mechanism of action and almost every component of the immune system is involved: IVIG interferes with costimulatory molecules, suppresses antibody production, hinders complement activation and MAC formation, and modulates the expression of Fc receptors on macrophages and diminishes chemokine, cytokine and adhesion molecule synthesis.[87]

The indications for the use of IVIG in MG are identical as with PLEX. The induction dose is 2 g/kg divided over 2 to 5 days (see **Table1**), but typically we do the induction over 2 to 3 days, unless the patient is hospitalized. A variety of complications have been reported with the use of IVIG in neuromuscular diseases, but most are mild to moderate in severity.[88] Prospective studies of IVIG use in neuromuscular disease have shown that headache is common, but that the incidence of serious adverse events is minimal.[74] Acute renal failure is uncommon and related to patient dehydration and the prior use of sucrose or maltose diluents. Other severe and rare reactions are anaphylaxis, stroke, myocardial infarction, deep venous thrombosis, and pulmonary emboli.

ECULIZUMAB

Complement has been known to have a crucial role in the pathogenesis of MG,[89–91] leading to the hypothesis that inhibiting various stages of the complement cascade could lead to clinical improvement in MG. Eculizumab is a recombinant humanized monoclonal antibody that binds to the C5 complement protein and inhibits its subsequent cleavage and formation of the C5b-9 membrane attack complex. It was recently approved in late 2017 for the treatment of adult patients with generalized MG who are AChR antibody–positive after successful trials.[92] Candidates for this novel therapy are those in a moderate/severe status category despite receiving adequate trials with most if not all of the discussed immunotherapies. The drug is given via intravenous infusion with a recommended dosage regimen of 900 mg/wk for the first 4 weeks, 1200 mg for the fifth week, and 1200 mg every 2 weeks thereafter (see **Table 1**). Eculizumab requires meningococcal vaccination before starting therapy. The introduction of complement inhibition could dramatically change how we manage patients with MG. Other drugs that inhibit complements are currently under study for MG.

SURGICAL TREATMENT: THYMECTOMY

Thymectomy has a central role in the treatment of MG. In thymomatous MG, the tumor should be removed. Tumor histologic grade, excision margins, and any distal spread guide treatment decisions regarding any subsequent radiation, chemotherapy, and monitoring. Along with thymoma, the entirety of the thymus tissue should be removed. Improvement in myasthenic symptoms may or may not follow. In multimorbid patients with high operative risk, palliative radiation therapy as an alternate can also be considered.[22]

In nonthymomatous generalized MG, thymectomy has become the standard despite a lack of evidence from a good prospective clinical trial. Two systematic reviews of the existing thymectomy literature emphasized this knowledge gap and recommended the MG field perform a randomized, controlled trial.[93–95] However, owing to the difficulty of performing controlled trials involving thoracic surgery in a rare disease, high-quality evidence about thymectomy had been lacking. A recently completed landmark international, randomized, rater-blinded clinical trial controlling for medical treatment was designed to address this uncertainty.[96] One hundred twenty-six recently diagnosed patients, ages 18 through 65 with AChR antibody–positive generalized MG were randomized to receive either extended transsternal thymectomy plus prednisone versus medical management with prednisone. Over a 3-year follow-up period, the time-weighted average QMG score was lower in the patients who underwent thymectomy (6.15 vs 8.99; *P*<.001). Similarly, the thymectomy group had a lower time-weighted alternate-day prednisone dose requirement (initially reported at 44 mg vs 60 mg; *P*<.001), which was later corrected to 32 mg versus 54 mg (95% confidence interval, 12–32 mg; *P*<.001) **Fig. 2**. Also in the thymectomy group, there were fewer patients requiring additional immunosuppression, fewer adverse events, and fewer admissions for myasthenic crises.

These data provide support for thymectomy as a first-line treatment modality that can improve MG status and decrease the required dose and duration of immunotherapy in generalized MG. The operation should be scheduled when the patient is neurologically optimized, because perioperative events can exacerbate myasthenic weakness. Patients with persistent bulbar, respiratory, or limb weakness should be treated with PLEX before surgery. Surprisingly, the effects of the thymectomy could be observed as early as 3 to 4 months and were maintained for the entire 3-year study.

Thymectomy in MuSK, LRP4, and agrin antibody–positive patients is not supported by current evidence.[22] Patients with MG with MuSK antibodies were not included in the recent thymectomy study. Nevertheless, MuSK and "double-negative" antibody patients have undergone thymectomy and have done well.[14] Similarly, there is limited evidence to support thymectomy in patients with ocular MG, although if the patient is AChR antibody positive, it may be considered in refractory cases.[97]

The recently completed thymectomy trial mandated a sternal-splitting procedure. Several new less invasive procedures are now being used for thymus removal (**Table 3**). Video-assisted thoracoscopic surgery and robotic approaches to thymectomy such as robotic video-assisted thoracoscopic surgery offer shorter hospital durations of stay and limited morbidity have emerged as alternatives to the classic

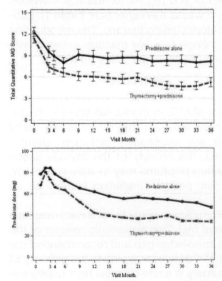

QMG Score (Mean±SE) by Treatment Group

- **QMG difference: 2.85 pts (99.5% CI 0.47–5.22; *P*<.001)**

Time-Weighted Average AD Prednisone Dose (Mean±SE) by Treatment Group

- **Prednisone dose difference:32 mg vs 54 mg (95% CI 12–32 mg; *P*<.001)**

Fig. 2. Wolfe et al thymectomy in MG. (*Data from* New England Journal of Medicine 2016;375(6):511–522.)

Table 3 Thymectomy Procedures	
Type	**Year**
Sternal splitting	Early 1900s
Maximally invasive	1980s
Transcervical	1988
Video-assisted thoracoscopic surgery	Late 1990s
Robotics (DaVinci)	Early 2000s

transsternal approach.[98,99] There are no trials comparing these surgical techniques, however, and available reports suggest comparable results.

TREATMENT STRATEGIES FOR GENERALIZED MYASTHENIA GRAVIS

The vast majority of patients with MG improve with therapy over time. Some can often go into remission or minimal manifestation status.[100] For refractory patients, obtaining care in specialized centers is likely particularly beneficial. A complete remission is defined as having no symptoms or signs and being off all medications for 2 years. Pharmacologic remission is also no symptoms or signs for 2 years, but on stable medication doses. Minimal manifestation status indicates no symptoms, but includes minimal clinical signs such as mild orbicularis oculi or hip flexor weakness (which may never fully resolve).

Fig. 3A summarizes our suggested treatment algorithm for generalized MG. First-line treatment is acetylcholinesterase inhibitors. Simultaneously, the patient should be considered for thymectomy. If a patient remains symptomatic on pyridostigmine, then it is probably time to initiate corticosteroid therapy. We consider acetylcholinesterase inhibitors, corticosteroids, and thymectomy all first-line therapies for generalized MG.

All newly diagnosed patients with MG should have a chest computed tomography scan to assess for thymoma. For patients with thymoma, thymectomy should be done immediately or as soon as the patient is strong enough after initiating immunomodulatory treatment to undergo surgery. We want to emphasize that the chest computed tomography scan is done to search for thymoma and not for thymic "hyperplasia" to decide if a thymectomy should be done in nonthymomatous patients. The decision for thymectomy in nonthymomatous patient is not based on the results of the chest computed tomography scan.

If the patient does not progress to a minimal manifestation status or remission, additional immune therapy should be considered until disease control is attained. Typically, patients with generalized disease require pyridostigmine with prednisone for the initial control of their disease, because pyridostigmine is not enough. For patients with severe weakness at presentation, or if they are diabetic, a steroid-sparing agent such as azathioprine may be started simultaneously with prednisone. If the patient worsens after a prednisone taper, second-line immunosuppressive therapy with azathioprine can be added at that time, realizing that the full benefit of azathioprine therapy may not occur for 12 to 18 months. If an agent that works faster is preferred, then IVIG or cyclosporine (or tacrolimus) are the other second-line choices that have been shown to be effective in randomized, controlled trials (**Table 4**). We use IVIG as a second-line immunosuppressive agent and usually in a patient who has improved but still has symptoms and signs of MG. We do not

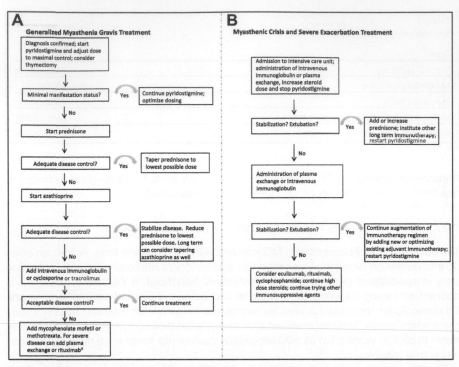

Fig. 3. Suggested algorithms for the treatment of generalized myasthenia gravis and myasthenic crisis. (*A*) Generalized myasthenia gravis treatment. (*B*) Myasthenic crisis and severe exacerbation treatment. [a] If not better, consider eculizumab.

Table 4
Treatment recommendations for myasthenia gravis

Prior to 2007	2018
1st Line	
Tensilon®	Enlon®
Pyridostigmine	Pyridostigmine
Prednisone	Prednisone
Thymectomy?	Thymectomy! YES
2nd Line	
Azathioprine	Azathioprine
Mycophenolate mofetil	Cyclosporine/tacrolimus
Cyclosporine	IVIG
3rd Line	
IVIG	Plasma exchange
Plasma exchange	Mycophenolate mofetil
	Methotrexate
4th Line	
None	Eculizumab (Soliris®)
	Rituximab
5th Line	
None	Cyclophosphamide

use IVIG as a first-line treatment, although the results of ongoing trials of IVIG could alter our practice. Third- and fourth-line options are plasmapheresis, mycophenolate mofetil, methotrexate, and rituximab, and can be used subsequently. In patients who have not responded to these therapies, we discuss chronic therapy with eculizumab infusions every other week.

At this time, we are considering eculizumab use in patients who are on prednisone and have tried 1 or more additional immunosuppressive drugs with incomplete disease control. In part, this decision is based on not having enough experience with the drug in our clinics and in part owing to the significant expense of the drug. Interestingly and surprisingly the US Food and Drug Administration approved labeling indication is for generalized MG with no requirement that the patient is on any other immunosuppressant therapy.

There are limited trial data to guide tapering of immune therapies in patients who have attained minimal manifestation status or pharmacologic remission. High-dose corticosteroid therapy started early in the course of MG should be considered for tapering 1 to 2 months after the patient has begun to improve. The goal is to try to get patients off prednisone if possible after 1 year or so of therapy. Sometimes, this maneuver is possible, but sometimes patients need to be left on a small dose of prednisone to prevent a relapse such as 5 to 7.5 mg/d or every other day. This determination can only be made by trial and error. After the patient has tapered off prednisone, then the steroid-sparing agents can also be tapered. Generally, we try to taper off prednisone first, leaving the patient on the second agent for a period of time (a year or two) before we attempt to slowly taper off the steroid-sparing agent.

TREATMENT STRATEGIES FOR MYASTHENIC CRISIS

MGFA grade 5 is a myasthenic crisis in which a patient is on mechanical ventilation. For patients in impending crises requiring intubation, abnormal blood gas levels cannot be relied on because they are insufficiently sensitive to impeding respiratory failure. Owing to the nature of myasthenic fatigability, clinical decline can be rapid and unexpected. Patients should be closely monitored for paradoxic breathing, orthopnea, diaphoresis, and a decline in pulmonary function via vital capacity and negative inspiratory force testing.

The treatment of MG crisis consists of rapid immunotherapy with either IVIG or PLEX. Concurrently, patients should be evaluated for infection and other precipitating events, such as the use of medications that can exacerbate MG. Because the effects of IVIG or PLEX are limited to several weeks, long-term immunosuppression should be intensified simultaneously and most frequently with prednisone, up to 100 mg/d or the methylprednisolone intravenous equivalent. Although acetylcholinesterase inhibitors are available intravenously, they should not be given in the setting of a crisis because they can increase respiratory secretions and complicate airway management. Therefore, all acetylcholinesterase inhibitors are stopped while the patient is intubated. This step is not because of the possibility of cholinergic crisis, which, as we stated, does not occur in the modern era with routinely used does of acetylcholinesterase inhibitors.

We do not have optimal data on the use of IVIG versus PLEX in myasthenic crisis. Gajdos and colleagues in France[85,86] and then Bril and colleagues in Canada[62] performed comparative effectiveness studies of IVIG and PLEX in moderate and severe MG and found the treatments to be equivalent. However, a few of these patients were in actual crises on a ventilator. A small controlled cross-over study of IVIG and PLEX showed similar efficacy in MG but faster onset of improvement at 1 week with

Table 5
Advantages and disadvantages of IVIG versus PLEX in MG

Pro-PLEX	Con-PLEX	Pro-IVIG	Con-IVIG
Probably effective	No RCT	Positive RCT	Insurance coverage limitations; not FDA approved for MG
Longer track record	Morbidity; need for central access	Ease of use	Shorter track record
May work faster	Sophisticated equipment; need for trained staff	Generally well-tolerated	Rare side effects: anaphylaxis, kidney injury, thrombosis

Abbreviations: FDA, US Food and Drug Administration; IVIG, intravenous immunoglobulin; MG, myasthenia gravis; PLEX, plasma exchange; RCT, randomized, controlled trial.

PLEX.[101] In addition, a retrospective study in juvenile MG showed a more consistent response to PLEX that IVIG.[78] The selection between these treatments often depends on availability and institutional experience in addition to individual patient factors. **Fig. 3**B summarizes our suggested treatment algorithm for myasthenic crisis. The pros and cons of IVIG versus PLEX are shown in **Table 5**.

Once a patient is on a ventilator, typically they need to be mechanically ventilated for 5 to 7 days. Extubating a patient after only a few days of mechanical ventilation often results in reintubation. Therefore, a conservative approach to extubation is recommended in this setting.

Emerging Therapies

There are other drugs that inhibit complement currently under study for MG. A phase II industry trial of belumimab, a monoclonal antibody against B-cell activating factor, was just completed with results pending. A multicenter investigator initiated subcutaneous gamma globulin study in MG (NCT02100969) is underway with the University of Kansas as the primary organizing site. A phase II study with a drug that increases muscle contractions, tirasemtiv, to improve strength in patients with MG was recently completed with some encouraging results.[102] As noted, the results of the National Institutes of Health–funded rituximab study in generalized MG will be released in 2018 (NCT02110706).

REFERENCES

1. Deenen JC, Horlings CG, Verschuuren JJ, et al. The epidemiology of neuromuscular disorders: a comprehensive overview of the literature. J Neuromuscul Dis 2015;2(1):73–85.
2. Walker MB. Treatment of myasthenia gravis with physostigmine. Lancet 1934; 223(5779):1200–1.
3. Grob D, Brunner N, Namba T, et al. Lifetime course of myasthenia gravis. Muscle Nerve 2008;37(2):141–9.
4. Carr AS, Cardwell CR, McCarron PO, et al. A systematic review of population based epidemiological studies in myasthenia gravis. BMC Neurol 2010;10:46.
5. Proudfoot A. The early toxicology of physostigmine: a tale of beans, great men and egos. Toxicol Rev 2006;25(2):99–138.
6. Walker MB. The James Lind Library: treatment of myasthenia with Physostigmine. Video of original Mary Walker patient treated with physostigmine. 1934.

Available at: http://www.jameslindlibrary.org/walker-mb-1934/. Accessed June 13, 2017.

7. Walker M. Case showing the effect of prostigmin on myasthenia gravis. Proc R Soc Med 1935;28:759–61.

8. Osserman KE, Teng P, Kaplan LI. Studies in myasthenia gravis; preliminary report on therapy with mestinon bromide. J Am Med Assoc 1954;155(11):961–5.

9. Schwab RS, Timberlake WH. Pyridostigmin (mestinon) in the treatment of myasthenia gravis. N Engl J Med 1954;251(7):271–2.

10. Tether JE. Mestinon in myasthenia gravis; preliminary report. Dis Nerv Syst 1954;15(8):227–31.

11. Westerberg MR, Magee KR. Mestinon in the treatment of myasthenia gravis. Neurology 1954;4(10):762–72.

12. Hatanaka Y, Hemmi S, Morgan MB, et al. Nonresponsiveness to anticholinesterase agents in patients with MuSK-antibody-positive MG. Neurology 2005; 65(9):1508–9.

13. Pasnoor M, Wolfe GI, Nations S, et al. Clinical findings in MuSK-antibody positive myasthenia gravis: a U.S. experience. Muscle Nerve 2010;41(3):370–4.

14. VanderPluym J, Vajsar J, Jacob FD, et al. Clinical characteristics of pediatric myasthenia: a surveillance study. Pediatrics 2013;132(4):e939–944.

15. Kupersmith MJ, Ying G. Ocular motor dysfunction and ptosis in ocular myasthenia gravis: effects of treatment. Br J Ophthalmol 2005;89(10):1330–4.

16. Mittal MK, Barohn RJ, Pasnoor M, et al. Ocular myasthenia gravis in an academic neuro-ophthalmology clinic: clinical features and therapeutic response. J Clin Neuromuscul Dis 2011;13(1):46–52.

17. Warmolts JR, Engel WK. Benefit from alternate-day prednisone in myasthenia gravis. N Engl J Med 1972;286(1):17–20.

18. Jenkins RB. Treatment of myasthenia gravis with prednisone. Lancet 1972; 1(7754):765–7.

19. Pascuzzi RM, Coslett HB, Johns TR. Long-term corticosteroid treatment of myasthenia gravis: report of 116 patients. Ann Neurol 1984;15(3):291–8.

20. Benatar M, McDermott MP, Sanders DB, et al. Efficacy of prednisone for the treatment of ocular myasthenia (EPITOME): a randomized, controlled trial. Muscle Nerve 2016;53(3):363–9.

21. Lindberg C, Andersen O, Lefvert AK. Treatment of myasthenia gravis with methylprednisolone pulse: a double blind study. Acta Neurol Scand 1998;97(6): 370–3.

22. Sanders DB, Wolfe GI, Benatar M, et al. International consensus guidance for management of myasthenia gravis: executive summary. Neurology 2016; 87(4):419–25.

23. Gilhus NE. Myasthenia gravis. N Engl J Med 2016;375(26):2570–81.

24. Seybold ME, Drachman DB. Gradually increasing doses of prednisone in myasthenia gravis. Reducing the hazards of treatment. N Engl J Med 1974;290(2): 81–4.

25. A trial of mycophenolate mofetil with prednisone as initial immunotherapy in myasthenia gravis. Neurology 2008;71(6):394–9.

26. Benatar M, Kaminski HJ. Evidence report: the medical treatment of ocular myasthenia (an evidence-based review): report of the Quality Standards Subcommittee of the American Academy of Neurology. Neurology 2007;68(24):2144–9.

27. Kupersmith MJ, Latkany R, Homel P. Development of generalized disease at 2 years in patients with ocular myasthenia gravis. Arch Neurol 2003;60(2):243–8.

28. Monsul NT, Patwa HS, Knorr AM, et al. The effect of prednisone on the progression from ocular to generalized myasthenia gravis. J Neurol Sci 2004;217(2): 131–3.

29. Barohn RD, Dimachkie MM. Immunomodulatory therapies in myasthenia gravis. In: Mazia C, editor. Miastenia gravis y trastornos relacionados. Buenos Aires (Argentina): Editorial Inter-Medica; 2017. p. 273–88.

30. Mertens HG, Hertel G, Reuther P, et al. Effect of immunosuppressive drugs (azathioprine). Ann N Y Acad Sci 1981;377:691–9.

31. Witte AS, Cornblath DR, Parry GJ, et al. Azathioprine in the treatment of myasthenia gravis. Ann Neurol 1984;15(6):602–5.

32. Palace J, Newsom-Davis J, Lecky B. A randomized double-blind trial of prednisolone alone or with azathioprine in myasthenia gravis. Myasthenia Gravis Study Group. Neurology 1998;50(6):1778–83.

33. Mantegazza R, Antozzi C, Peluchetti D, et al. Azathioprine as a single drug or in combination with steroids in the treatment of myasthenia gravis. J Neurol 1988; 235(8):449–53.

34. Sommer N, Sigg B, Melms A, et al. Ocular myasthenia gravis: response to long-term immunosuppressive treatment. J Neurol Neurosurg Psychiatry 1997;62(2): 156–62.

35. Hohlfeld R, Michels M, Heininger K, et al. Azathioprine toxicity during long-term immunosuppression of generalized myasthenia gravis. Neurology 1988;38(2): 258–61.

36. Bernatsky S, Clarke AE, Suissa S. Hematologic malignant neoplasms after drug exposure in rheumatoid arthritis. Arch Intern Med 2008;168(4):378–81.

37. Booth RA, Ansari MT, Loit E, et al. Assessment of thiopurine S-methyltransferase activity in patients prescribed thiopurines: a systematic review. Ann Intern Med 2011;154(12):814–23, w-295-818.

38. Simmons WD, Rayhill SC, Sollinger HW. Preliminary risk-benefit assessment of mycophenolate mofetil in transplant rejection. Drug Saf 1997;17(2):75–92.

39. Hauser RA, Malek AR, Rosen R. Successful treatment of a patient with severe refractory myasthenia gravis using mycophenolate mofetil. Neurology 1998; 51(3):912–3.

40. Chaudhry V, Cornblath DR, Griffin JW, et al. Mycophenolate mofetil: a safe and promising immunosuppressant in neuromuscular diseases. Neurology 2001; 56(1):94–6.

41. Meriggioli MN, Ciafaloni E, Al-Hayk KA, et al. Mycophenolate mofetil for myasthenia gravis: an analysis of efficacy, safety, and tolerability. Neurology 2003; 61(10):1438–40.

42. Sanders DB, Hart IK, Mantegazza R, et al. An international, phase III, randomized trial of mycophenolate mofetil in myasthenia gravis. Neurology 2008;71(6): 400–6.

43. Hehir MK, Burns TM, Alpers J, et al. Mycophenolate mofetil in AChR-antibody-positive myasthenia gravis: outcomes in 102 patients. Muscle Nerve 2010;41(5): 593–8.

44. Mycophenolate REMS risks of first trimester pregnancy loss and congenital malformations. Available at: https://www.mycophenolaterems.com/. Accessed January 18, 2018.

45. Vernino S, Salomao DR, Habermann TM, et al. Primary CNS lymphoma complicating treatment of myasthenia gravis with mycophenolate mofetil. Neurology 2005;65(4):639–41.

46. Dubal DB, Mueller S, Ruben BS, et al. T-cell lymphoproliferative disorder following mycophenolate treatment for myasthenia gravis. Muscle Nerve 2009; 39(6):849–50.
47. Tindall RS, Rollins JA, Phillips JT, et al. Preliminary results of a double-blind, randomized, placebo-controlled trial of cyclosporine in myasthenia gravis. N Engl J Med 1987;316(12):719–24.
48. Tindall RS, Phillips JT, Rollins JA, et al. A clinical therapeutic trial of cyclosporine in myasthenia gravis. Ann N Y Acad Sci 1993;681:539–51.
49. Ciafaloni E, Nikhar NK, Massey JM, et al. Retrospective analysis of the use of cyclosporine in myasthenia gravis. Neurology 2000;55(3):448–50.
50. Nagane Y, Utsugisawa K, Obara D, et al. Efficacy of low-dose FK506 in the treatment of Myasthenia gravis–a randomized pilot study. Eur Neurol 2005;53(3): 146–50.
51. Liu C, Gui M, Cao Y, et al. Tacrolimus improves symptoms of children with myasthenia gravis refractory to prednisone. Pediatr Neurol 2017;77:42–7.
52. Brown PM, Pratt AG, Isaacs JD. Mechanism of action of methotrexate in rheumatoid arthritis, and the search for biomarkers. Nat Rev Rheumatol 2016; 12(12):731–42.
53. Heckmann JM, Rawoot A, Bateman K, et al. A single-blinded trial of methotrexate versus azathioprine as steroid-sparing agents in generalized myasthenia gravis. BMC Neurol 2011;11:97.
54. Pasnoor M, He J, Herbelin L, et al. A randomized controlled trial of methotrexate for patients with generalized myasthenia gravis. Neurology 2016;87(1):57–64.
55. Perez MC, Buot WL, Mercado-Danguilan C, et al. Stable remissions in myasthenia gravis. Neurology 1981;31(1):32–7.
56. De Feo LG, Schottlender J, Martelli NA, et al. Use of intravenous pulsed cyclophosphamide in severe, generalized myasthenia gravis. Muscle Nerve 2002; 26(1):31–6.
57. Drachman DB, Jones RJ, Brodsky RA. Treatment of refractory myasthenia: "rebooting" with high-dose cyclophosphamide. Ann Neurol 2003;53(1):29–34.
58. Tandan R, Hehir MK 2nd, Waheed W, et al. Rituximab treatment of myasthenia gravis: a systematic review. Muscle Nerve 2017;56(2):185–96.
59. Zaja F, Russo D, Fuga G, et al. Rituximab for myasthenia gravis developing after bone marrow transplant. Neurology 2000;55(7):1062–3.
60. Vander Heiden JA, Stathopoulos P, Zhou JQ, et al. Dysregulation of B cell repertoire formation in myasthenia gravis patients revealed through deep sequencing. J Immunol 2017;198(4):1460–73.
61. Collongues N, Casez O, Lacour A, et al. Rituximab in refractory and non-refractory myasthenia: a retrospective multicenter study. Muscle Nerve 2012; 46(5):687–91.
62. Hain B, Jordan K, Deschauer M, et al. Successful treatment of MuSK antibody-positive myasthenia gravis with rituximab. Muscle Nerve 2006;33(4):575–80.
63. Diaz-Manera J, Martinez-Hernandez E, Querol L, et al. Long-lasting treatment effect of rituximab in MuSK myasthenia. Neurology 2012;78(3):189–93.
64. Silvestri NJ, Wolfe GI. Myasthenia gravis. Semin Neurol 2012;32(3):215–26.
65. Kanth KM, Solorzano GE, Goldman MD. PML in a patient with myasthenia gravis treated with multiple immunosuppressing agents. Neurol Clin Pract 2016;6(2): e17–9.
66. Vermeer NS, Straus SM, Mantel-Teeuwisse AK, et al. Drug-induced progressive multifocal leukoencephalopathy: lessons learned from contrasting natalizumab and rituximab. Clin Pharmacol Ther 2015;98(5):542–50.

67. Nowak R, Coffey C, Goldstein J, et al. A phase 2 trial of rituximab in myasthenia gravis: study update. 14th International Congress on Neuromuscular Diseases (ICNMD XIV). Toronto (Canada), July 7, 2016.
68. Pinching AJ, Peters DK. Remission of myasthenia gravis following plasma-exchange. Lancet 1976;2(8000):1373–6.
69. Dau PC, Lindstrom JM, Cassel CK, et al. Plasmapheresis and immunosuppressive drug therapy in myasthenia gravis. N Engl J Med 1977;297(21):1134–40.
70. Plasmapheresis and acute Guillain-Barre syndrome. The Guillain-Barre syndrome Study Group. Neurology 1985;35(8):1096–104.
71. Patwa HS, Chaudhry V, Katzberg H, et al. Evidence-based guideline: intravenous immunoglobulin in the treatment of neuromuscular disorders: report of the Therapeutics and Technology Assessment Subcommittee of the American Academy of Neurology. Neurology 2012;78(13):1009–15.
72. Gajdos P, Chevret S, Toyka K. Plasma exchange for myasthenia gravis. Cochrane Database Syst Rev 2002;(4):CD002275.
73. Barth D, Nabavi Nouri M, Ng E, et al. Comparison of IVIg and PLEX in patients with myasthenia gravis. Neurology 2011;76(23):2017–23.
74. Zinman L, Ng E, Bril V. IV immunoglobulin in patients with myasthenia gravis: a randomized controlled trial. Neurology 2007;68(11):837–41.
75. Ebadi H, Barth D, Bril V. Safety of plasma exchange therapy in patients with myasthenia gravis. Muscle Nerve 2013;47(4):510–4.
76. Yeh JH, Wang SH, Chien PJ, et al. Changes in serum cytokine levels during plasmapheresis in patients with myasthenia gravis. Eur J Neurol 2009;16(12):1318–22.
77. Mandawat A, Mandawat A, Kaminski HJ, et al. Outcome of plasmapheresis in myasthenia gravis: delayed therapy is not favorable. Muscle Nerve 2011;43(4):578–84.
78. Liew WK, Powell CA, Sloan SR, et al. Comparison of plasmapheresis and intravenous immunoglobulin as maintenance therapies for juvenile myasthenia gravis. JAMA Neurol 2014;71(5):575–80.
79. Shemin D, Briggs D, Greenan M. Complications of therapeutic plasma exchange: a prospective study of 1,727 procedures. J Clin Apher 2007;22(5):270–6.
80. Ahmed F, Vamanan K, Dimachkie M, et al. Arteriovenous fistula venous access for long-term outpatient plasma exchange for neuromuscular disorders. American Academy of Neurology Annual Meeting. Seattle (WA), April 25 - May 02, 2009.
81. Gajdos P, Outin H, Elkharrat D, et al. High-dose intravenous gammaglobulin for myasthenia gravis. Lancet 1984;1(8373):406–7.
82. Arsura EL, Bick A, Brunner NG, et al. High-dose intravenous immunoglobulin in the management of myasthenia gravis. Arch Intern Med 1986;146(7):1365–8.
83. Achiron A, Barak Y, Miron S, et al. Immunoglobulin treatment in refractory myasthenia gravis. Muscle Nerve 2000;23(4):551–5.
84. Wolfe GI, Barohn RJ, Foster BM, et al. Randomized, controlled trial of intravenous immunoglobulin in myasthenia gravis. Muscle Nerve 2002;26(4):549–52.
85. Gajdos P, Chevret S, Clair B, et al. Clinical trial of plasma exchange and high-dose intravenous immunoglobulin in myasthenia gravis. Myasthenia Gravis Clinical Study Group. Ann Neurol 1997;41(6):789–96.
86. Gajdos P, Tranchant C, Clair B, et al. Treatment of myasthenia gravis exacerbation with intravenous immunoglobulin: a randomized double-blind clinical trial. Arch Neurol 2005;62(11):1689–93.

87. Dalakas MC. Intravenous immunoglobulin in autoimmune neuromuscular diseases. JAMA 2004;291(19):2367–75.
88. Brannagan TH 3rd, Nagle KJ, Lange DJ, et al. Complications of intravenous immune globulin treatment in neurologic disease. Neurology 1996;47(3):674–7.
89. Barohn RJ, Brey RL. Soluble terminal complement components in human myasthenia gravis. Clin Neurol Neurosurg 1993;95(4):285–90.
90. Engel AG, Arahata K. The membrane attack complex of complement at the end-plate in myasthenia gravis. Ann N Y Acad Sci 1987;505:326–32.
91. Engel AG, Lambert EH, Howard FM. Immune complexes (IgG and C3) at the motor end-plate in myasthenia gravis: ultrastructural and light microscopic localization and electrophysiologic correlations. Mayo Clin Proc 1977;52(5): 267–80.
92. Howard JF Jr, Barohn RJ, Cutter GR, et al. A randomized, double-blind, placebo-controlled phase II study of eculizumab in patients with refractory generalized myasthenia gravis. Muscle Nerve 2013;48(1):76–84.
93. Gronseth GS, Barohn RJ. Practice parameter: thymectomy for autoimmune myasthenia gravis (an evidence-based review): report of the Quality Standards Subcommittee of the American Academy of Neurology. Neurology 2000;55(1): 7–15.
94. Cea G, Benatar M, Verdugo RJ, et al. Thymectomy for non-thymomatous myasthenia gravis. Cochrane Database Syst Rev 2013;(10):CD008111.
95. Kissel JT, Franklin GM. Treatment of myasthenia gravis: a call to arms. Neurology 2000;55(1):3–4.
96. Wolfe GI, Kaminski HJ, Aban IB, et al. Randomized trial of thymectomy in myasthenia gravis. N Engl J Med 2016;375(6):511–22.
97. Skeie GO, Apostolski S, Evoli A, et al. Guidelines for treatment of autoimmune neuromuscular transmission disorders. Eur J Neurol 2010;17(7):893–902.
98. Goldstein SD, Culbertson NT, Garrett D, et al. Thymectomy for myasthenia gravis in children: a comparison of open and thoracoscopic approaches. J Pediatr Surg 2015;50(1):92–7.
99. Wagner AJ, Cortes RA, Strober J, et al. Long-term follow-up after thymectomy for myasthenia gravis: thoracoscopic vs open. J Pediatr Surg 2006;41(1):50–4 [discussion: 50–4].
100. Jaretzki A 3rd, Barohn RJ, Ernstoff RM, et al. Myasthenia gravis: recommendations for clinical research standards. Task Force of the Medical Scientific Advisory Board of the Myasthenia Gravis Foundation of America. Neurology 2000; 55(1):16–23.
101. Ronager J, Ravnborg M, Hermansen I, et al. Immunoglobulin treatment versus plasma exchange in patients with chronic moderate to severe myasthenia gravis. Artif Organs 2001;25(12):967–73.
102. Sanders DB, Rosenfeld J, Dimachkie MM, et al. A double-blinded, randomized, placebo-controlled trial to evaluate efficacy, safety, and tolerability of single doses of tirasemtiv in patients with acetylcholine receptor-binding antibody-positive myasthenia gravis. Neurotherapeutics 2015;12(2):455–60.

Measuring Clinical Treatment Response in Myasthenia Gravis

Carolina Barnett, MD, PhD[a,1,*], Laura Herbelin, BSc, CCRP[b],
Mazen M. Dimachkie, MD[b], Richard J. Barohn, MD[b]

KEYWORDS

- Myasthenia gravis • Outcome measurement • Responsiveness
- Minimal important difference • Disability

KEY POINTS

- Newer outcome measures incorporate more input from patients and have undergone more rigorous psychometric analysis.
- Ideal measures in clinical care are brief to administer, whereas in clinical trials more comprehensive and overlapping measures are needed to demonstrate a positive effect.
- Minimal clinically important differences are available in very few of the outcome measures but can help to inform clinical trial design and sample size estimation.

INTRODUCTION TO HEALTH-RELATED OUTCOME MEASURES

There are several aspects of health that can be measured, and these represent different aspects of the disease, from the pathophysiology (eg, antibody titers), to the symptoms

Disclosure Statement: C. Barnett participated in the development of the Myasthenia Gravis Impairment Index (MGII) and might receive royalties in the future. She has provided consultancy to UCB regarding outcomes for myasthenia gravis studies. Dr R. Barohn is on the speaker's bureau for NuFactor, Grifols Therapeutics Inc, and Plan 365 Inc. He is on the advisory board for CSL Behring GmbH, and has received an honorarium from Option Care. He has received research grants from the NIH, FDA/OOPD, NINDS, Novartis, Sanofi/Genzyme, Biomarin, IONIS, Teva, Cytocenetics, Eli Lilly, and PTC. Dr M. Dimachkie is on the speaker's bureau or is a consultant for Alnylam, Baxalta, Catalyst, CSL-Behring, Mallinckrodt, Novartis, and NuFactor. He has also received grants from Alexion, Biomarin, Catalyst, CSL-Behring, the FDA/OPD, GSK, Grifols, MDA, the NIH, Novartis, Sanofi, and TMA. This work was supported by a CTSA grant from NCATS awarded to the University of Kansas for Frontiers: University of Kansas Clinical and Translational Science Institute (# UL1TR002366) The contents are solely the responsibility of the authors and do not necessarily represent the official views of the NIH or NCATS.
[a] Neurology (Medicine), University of Toronto, University Health Network, Toronto, Ontario, Canada; [b] Department of Neurology, University of Kansas Medical Center, 3901 Rainbow Boulevard, Kansas City, KS 66160, USA
[1] Present address: 200 Elizabeth Street, 5EC Room 322, Toronto, Ontario M5G 2C4, Canada.
* Corresponding author. 200 Elizabeth Street, 5EC Room 322, Toronto, Ontario M5G 2C4, Canada.
E-mail address: c.barnetttapia@utoronto.ca

and signs, to the effect on the individual and their relation to society.[1] Because different outcome measures are aimed at different aspects of the disease process, it is fundamental to understand what a given tool measures, as well as for which purpose it was developed and in which population it was tested. One way to understand these different aspects of the disease is through the International Classification of Functioning, Disability and Health (ICF),[2] published by the World Health Organization. The ICF identifies 3 major ways in which a disease or injury affects in individual: impairments of body function or structures, which are basically the signs and symptoms; activity limitations, which are the effects of the disease and its symptoms on activities of daily life; and participation limitations, which are the effects on a patient's social interactions, such as looking for work or caring for their family. Additionally, these aspects of the disease are also affected by personal and environmental factors (eg, social support, cultural factors, and accessibility). Disability is—according to the ICF—the interaction between symptoms, activities, and participation restrictions and personal and environmental factors.[2] Health-related quality of life (HRQoL) goes beyond the concept of disability and it is, by definition, a subjective and multidimensional concept, including physical functioning, mental or psychological well-being, occupational status, and social interactions.[3] The impairments of body functions/structures are thought to be less affected by social and environmental factors and, therefore, are typically considered to reflect more directly disease severity. This factor is why most outcome measures aimed at quantifying disease severity capture the signs and symptoms, whereas measures focused on the impact of the symptoms on the individual as a whole are usually disability or HRQoL measures. Putting these concepts into the perspective of a clinical trial, the primary outcome should match the study intervention. For example, a phase II study for a new medication will likely be focused on the effect of signs and symptoms, whereas a psychosocial intervention will probably have more effect on HRQoL or disability than on the symptoms in isolation. **Fig. 1** depicts the ICF model in relation to some of the outcome measures specific to myasthenia gravis (MG) that are available.

Additionally, when choosing an outcome measure, it is fundamental to recognize that, beyond what they measure, they might have been developed with different purposes, typically discriminative, predictive, and evaluative.[4] Discriminative means that a measure can distinguish between individuals that have different degrees of the underlying construct (eg, more or less severe disease). Predictive measures are aimed at classifying individuals such as in a diagnostic test or predicting an outcome. Finally, evaluative measures are aimed at detecting change, which is fundamental to determining treatment response. Additionally, there are several methodologic requirements that need to be met to ensure that the measure is adequate for the intended purpose. All measures have to be valid (ie, measure what they are supposed to measure) and reliable (ie, reproducible). In addition, evaluative measures have to demonstrate responsiveness, or the ability to detect change. To interpret change scores, it is important to know the minimal important difference (MID), which is the smallest change in a measure that is meaningful for patients.[5] Additionally, there has been a shift in recent years toward more patient-reported outcomes, considering that patients are the best judges of their disease status and that many symptoms or signs might not be evident in a clinical encounter or—when present—do not affect patient function. The specific standards for the development of outcome measures are beyond the scope of this article, but for those interested, the US Food and Drug Administration[6] and the COnsensus-based Standards for the selection of health Measurement INstruments (COSMIN)[7] guidelines are excellent resources. Finally, it is important to keep in mind that validity, reliability, and responsiveness are not universal characteristics of a measure, and depend on the populations and interventions tested.[8]

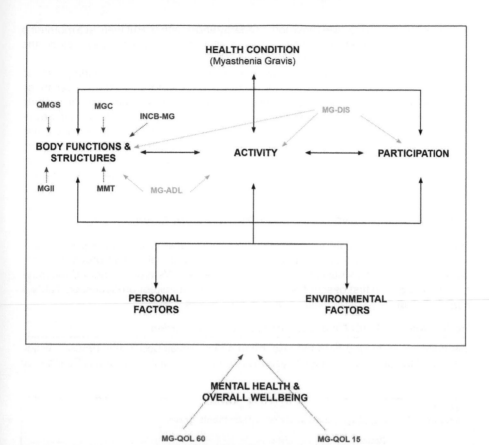

Fig. 1. Commonly Used myasthenia gravis (MG) outcomes in relation to the International Classification of Functioning, Disability and Health (ICF). The ICF framework (within the red box) and which aspects of the disease are measured by commonly used MG measures. Measures of health-related quality of life (HRQoL) also incorporate mental health and overall wellbeing. INCB-MG, Besta Neurologic Institute rating scale for MG; MG-ADL, Myasthenia Gravis Activities of Daily Living; MGC, Myasthenia Gravis Composite; MG-DIS, MG Disability Scale; MGII, Myasthenia Gravis Impairment Index; MMT, Manual Muscle Test; QMGS, Quantitative Myasthenia Gravis Score. (*Modified from* World Health Organization. International classification of functioning, disability and health (ICF). 1st edition. Geneva: World Health Organization; 2002.)

OUTCOME MEASUREMENT IN MYASTHENIA GRAVIS

MG presents specific challenges for outcome measurement. The classical manifestation of MG—fatigable weakness—results in signs and symptoms that fluctuate. These fluctuations can occur within the same day, because typically patients are more symptomatic as the day goes by, but also from day to day, and even within longer time-frames. Therefore, a clinical assessment that is anchored in a single time-point might be insufficient to cover the breadth of the manifestations of MG. In a qualitative study of patients' experiences with MG, patients consistently reported fatigability as a major manifestation of the disease.[9] Regarding the assessments, one patient said: "It's [the assessment] just such a quick snapshot of how I'm doing, really, at that very moment. And it seems so variable throughout the day. I could have a good hour where people wouldn't even know that I have MG at all. I look like I have lots of energy and whatnot. But then, at a moment's notice, it could completely change."[9] This is why many MG measures include the patients' report of their symptoms, or other measures of fatigability.[10–12]

There are several measures that have been used in MG studies, including generic measures, and reviewing all would not be feasible. Therefore, we only cover those measures that have been specifically developed for MG. Additionally, we only include measures that are available in English and where there are enough data on the development and validation process. To further organize the many MG-specific outcomes available, we have divided them by what they measure: signs and symptoms, and disability/HRQoL. Finally, we discuss other outcomes that are relevant for MG that do not directly fit into the disability framework, such as biomarkers and steroid-sparing effects.

MEASURES OF SIGNS AND SYMPTOMS OF MYASTHENIA GRAVIS

These measures constitute the majority of outcomes specifically developed for MG. For each measure, we provide a brief description of its development process, items, how it is scored, and its basic psychometric properties. We have organized the measures based on the first description of the measure or its direct predecessor. **Table 1** depicts the primary characteristics of these measures.

The Myasthenia Gravis Foundation of America Classification

This measure is derived from the Osserman score, developed in the 1950s,[13] which was one of the first classifications systems in MG. The Myasthenia Gravis Foundation

Table 1
Measures of signs and symptoms severity in myasthenia gravis

	Total Items	Patient Reported Items	Total Score	Interpretation	MID	Instrumentation
QMGS	13	0	0–39	Higher score, more severe disease	2 or 3 points	Spirometer, dynamometer
MMS	9	0	0–100	Lower score, more severe disease	NA	No
INCB-MG	11	2	0–427,153	Higher score, more severe disease	NA	No
MG-ADL	8	8	0–24	Higher score, more severe disease	2 points	No
MMT	30	0	0–120	Higher score, more severe disease	NA	No
MGC	10	4	0–50	Higher score, more severe disease	3 points	No
OBFR	5	0	0–21	Higher score, more severe disease	NA	Spirometer
MGII	28	22	0–84	Higher score, more severe disease	8.1 groups 5.5 individual	No

Abbreviations: INCB-MG, Besta Neurologic Institute rating scale for Myasthenia Gravis[29]; MG-ADL, Myasthenia Gravis Activities of Daily Living[19]; MGC, Myasthenia Gravis Composite[21]; MGII, Myasthenia Gravis Impairment Index[22]; MID, minimal important difference (these are for improvement); MMS, Myasthenia Muscle Score[57]; MMT, Manual Muscle Test[16]; NA, not applicable; OBFR, Oculo-bulbar Facial Respiratory Score[41]; QMGS, Quantitative Myasthenia Gravis Score.[10]

of America (MGFA) classification is aimed at separating patients in groups based on disease severity and the localization of the symptoms, and does not have an evaluative purpose. The MGFA classes are pure ocular (class I), mild generalized (class II), moderate generalized (class III), severe generalized (class IV), and intubation/myasthenic crisis (class V). Within the generalized categories II, III, and IV, patients are subclassified as class A if their symptoms are predominantly generalized or class B if their symptoms are predominantly bulbar.[14] The MGFA also has a system to classify patients based on postintervention outcomes and includes remission, defined as 1 year or longer without signs or symptoms and without any symptomatic (pyridostigmine) treatment, and which can be divided in complete (no pharmacologic treatment at all) or pharmacologic remission. Minimal manifestation status is defined as minimal signs or symptoms (no specific time-frame was defined) and pyridostigmine use may be accepted. Additionally, patients can be improved, unchanged, worse, experiencing an MG exacerbation, or have died of MG.[14] Because the original MGFA severity classification does not take into account those patients who are asymptomatic, many MG studies use a hybrid, whereby symptomatic patients are classified based on the I to V class system, and asymptomatic or oligosymptomatic patients are classified as remission or minimal manifestation status.[15]

The Quantitative Myasthenia Gravis Score

The Quantitative Myasthenia Gravis Score (QMGS) was developed in the context of a clinical trial in MG and originally had 8 items[16]; it was later modified for a trial of cyclosporine,[17] increasing the number of items to 13. This measure was modified again by Barohn and colleagues,[18] making the 13 items all based on the examination, and this is the version currently in use. The QMGS has several items that measure endurance or fatigability, taking into account the fluctuating nature of the disease. The items are as follows: ptosis, diplopia, orbicularis oculi weakness, swallowing a cup of water, speech, percent predicted forced vital capacity, grip strength (2 items), arm endurance (2 items), leg endurance (2 items), and neck flexion endurance. All items are scored on a scale of 0 to 3, and total scores range from 0 to 39; higher scores indicate greater disease severity. There are 2 studies on interobserver reliability[18,19] and one on test–retest reliability[20] showing adequate reliability coefficients. Construct validity has been studied by demonstrating correlations between the QMGS scores to other outcome measures like the Manual Muscle Test (MMT)[21] and Myasthenia Muscle Score,[19] as well as comparing QMGS scores across different MGFA classes, and with electrodiagnostic markers.[22] There is study on longitudinal validity where 53 patients were seen on a second visit between 2 and 10 months after initial examination. Using the physician's impression of change as marker or improvement, the difference in the QMGS score was significantly higher in those improved compared with those who were stable.[23]

The QMGS also has shown to be responsive to change in several clinical trials. In a randomized study of intravenous immunoglobulin (IVIG)[24] and in a cyclosporine trial,[17] treated patients had a statistically significant improvement in the QMGS compared with a placebo group. Based on the mean change in the cyclosporine trial and the reliability a studies, a change of greater than 3.5 points has been typically considered as significant.[17,18] Using the data from the IVIG versus placebo study, the MID with mild to moderate MG (QMGS $\leq$16) was calculated to be 2 points,[25] although patients with higher baseline values (QMGS >16) had a higher MID of 3 points, which is a well-described phenomenon. Additionally, the performance of the individual items of the QMGS was studied,[26] with evidence of floor effect—a high proportion of patients scoring 0 (best score) at baseline—on grip strength, dysarthria, swallowing, and percent forced vital capacity. The items that changed the most after treatment were ptosis, and arm, leg, and neck endurance. The main drawbacks of the QMGS are in terms of feasibility and ease of use, because it requires a dynamometer and spirometer and can take up to 25 minutes to complete. Therefore, it is mostly used in research rather than routine clinical assessments.

The Myasthenia Muscle Score

This measure was developed in the context of a clinical trial[27] and is extensively used in France. It has 9 items: 3 bulbar (chewing, swallowing, and speech), 1 ocular (combines diplopia and ptosis), 1 on eye closure, 2 axial muscles (neck flexors and sitting up), and 2 on limb endurance (arms/legs). All items are based on clinical examination, with maximal subscore values ranging from 10 to 15, and the total scores ranging from 0 to 100, with lower scores indicating greater disease severity. There is 1 small study on interobserver reliability, with an intraclass correlation coefficient (ICC) of 0.9, which is excellent.[19] There are no studies on test–retest reliability. Validity has been studied through correlations with the QMGS ($r = -0.87$)[19] in a small sample. The Myasthenia Muscle Score has been used as primary outcome in a trial of IVIG and plasma exchange,[28] and patients who received IVIG or plasma exchange improved by 16 points on average. However, there are no studies on the MID.

The Besta Neurologic Institute Rating Scale for Myasthenia Gravis

This measure was initially developed in 1988 for a clinical trial of azathioprine,[29] and has been used extensively in Italy. It was recently modified to improve the reliability of some items, as well as to remove the need for a spirometer or using a water test for swallowing.[30] The current version has 11 items: 1 ocular, 5 generalized, and 5 bulbar, all based on the physical examination, with the exception of the items on swallowing and breathing, which are based on the history. The scale is weighted, whereby bulbar items receive more weight than limb and ocular items—427,000 maximum points for bulbar/breathing problems and 153 maximum points for ocular and limb problems—and higher scores indicate more disease severity. The Besta Neurologic Institute rating scale for Myasthenia Gravis also includes 2 endurance tests: one of the arms and one of the legs, which are similar to the QMGS and measured in seconds. These measures are scored independently, rather than being factored into the total score. The total, bulbar, and generalized scores had good internal consistency (Cronbach's alpha = 0.79, 0.75, and 0.75, respectively), and good interrater reliability (kappa = 0.92).[30] Test–retest reliability was not described. In terms of construct validity, it has a high correlation with the MGC ($r = 0.83$). Responsiveness has not been formally assessed for the sum scores; however, the arm and leg endurance tests are responsive to change, confirming previous studies.[26,31]

The Myasthenia Gravis Activities of Daily Living

This instrument, like the modified QMGS, was developed for the trial of IVIG by Wolfe and colleagues.[32] This is a patient-reported outcome that combines 2 items on daily life activities—ability to brush teeth or comb hair, and limitations in the ability to rise from a chair—with 6 items reflecting other MG symptoms: diplopia, ptosis, chewing, swallowing, voice/speech problems, and respiratory symptoms.[10] Each item is scored between 0 and 3 and total scores range from 0 to 24, where higher scores indicate more disease severity. Test–retest reliability was demonstrated in 20 patients, with an ICC of 0.93.[33] Construct validity has been studied through correlations with the QMGS,[10] the Myasthenia Gravis Composite (MGC),[34] and the MG Quality of Life (MG-QOL)15,[33] showing moderate correlations with the QMGS ($r = 0.58$) and high with the MGC and MG-QOL15 (r = 0.85, 0.76). The responsiveness of the Myasthenia Gravis Activities of Daily Living (MG-ADL) was tested in a study of 76 patients who were assessed twice,[33] with variable interventions and time intervals between assessments. Patients were considered improved based on an improvement in a quality-of-life measure, the MG-QOL15,[35] and in the physician impression of change. The MID to classify an individual patient as a responder was 2 points—using a receiver operator characteristic curve approach—where the MID is the point of greatest sensitivity and specificity. The MG-ADL has been used in several clinical trials, including as a secondary outcome measure in the thymectomy randomized, controlled trial,[36] where treated patients and significantly greater improvement than those in the placebo arm (difference between groups, 1.17; P = .008). The main advantages of the MG-ADL are that it is very easy to use, and it is completely patient reported. A drawback is that it does not have a specific recall time frame (eg, 2 or 4 weeks) because it relies on comparing with the last visit, and that it is prone to floor effects.[12]

The Manual Muscle Test

This was developed in 2003,[21] with the aim of having a simple assessment of MG patients, without the need for instrumentation. The MMT evaluates the strength in 12 bilateral muscle groups and 6 ocular or axial (eg, neck flexors) muscles, that are usually affected in MG. Each muscle is scored from 0 (normal strength) to 4 (paralysis), and the total score is the sum of each muscle, where higher scores indicate more strength (less disease severity). Interrater reliability was assessed in 274 patients through Pearson's correlation, but ICCs were not reported.[21] Construct validity was tested through the correlations with the QMGS. The MMT has been used as secondary outcome measure in a clinical trial,[37] with low to moderate correlations (r = 0.30–0.59) between the change in MMT scores and change in the QMGS and the MG-ADL.[38] The MMT scores changed significantly after treatment (P<.001). Additionally, the MMT change scores were higher in those patients deemed improved (by physician impression of change) than in those who were unchanged. However, there are no studies on the MID. The main advantage of the MMT is the ease of use, because it is based on the routine neurologic examination. Drawbacks are that it measures static strength, so it is likely to be more affected by the natural fluctuations of the disease.

The Myasthenia Gravis Composite

The MGC was developed more recently, aiming for a simple yet comprehensive measure of MG severity. It was developed by combining items from other MG measures, based on their performance of 2 clinical trials of mycophenolate in MG.[37,39] The measures considered for items were the QMGS, the MG-ADL, and the MMT. Item selection was determined by responsiveness to treatment (defined by a positive physicians' and patients' impression of change), as well as with the correlations with the MG-QOL15, a disease-specific quality-of-life measure.[35] Final item selection and weights were decided by a large group of MG experts, and bulbar and generalized items have more weight than ocular items. The final measure has 10 items: 2 ocular (diplopia and ptosis) from the QMGS; 4 items (facial, neck, deltoids, and hip flexors strength) from the MMT, and 4 patient-reported items from the MG-ADL (chewing, swallowing, breathing, and speech). Regarding the latter, these are read to the patients and the whole scale is completed by an examiner. Total scores range from 0 to 50 where higher scores indicate greater disease severity. Interrater reliability was high in a study of 38 patients.[34] Construct validity was evaluated in 175 patients, and this was based on positive correlations between the MGC and other measures, including the MMT, ADL, and the MG-QOL15.[34] Responsiveness was studied in 151 patients who had routine follow-up examinations, with an average time between assessments of 4.7 months, and variable interventions within visits.[34] In that study, using a receiver operator characteristic curve and defining improvement based on the physician's impression of change and the change in the MG-QOL15, the MID for individuals was estimated at 3 points.[39] The MGC was recommended as the primary outcome measure of choice in MG trials by the MGFA scientific board,[40] and it has been subsequently used as primary or secondary outcome in several trials. The main strength of the MGC is its simplicity and the incorporation of the patient's history.

The Oculo-Bulbar Facial Score

This measure was developed specifically to quantify the signs and symptoms affecting the extraocular, facial, and respiratory muscles in MG, specifically considering patients with musculoskeletal MG.[41] The Oculo-Bulbar Facial Score has 1 item that sums the strength of 5 facial muscles, 1 item on palatal contractility, 1 on tongue appearance, 1 on forced vital capacity, and 1 on swallowing time, based on swallowing 100 mL of water. The total score ranges from 0 to 21, and higher scores indicate worse oculo-bulbar and respiratory function. A modified version removed 2 of the 5 facial muscles tested give low agreement between raters, and has a maximum possible score of 17.[41] Overall interrater reliability coefficients were not described. The Oculo-Bulbar Facial Score has moderate correlations with the MGC, MG-ADL, and MG-QoL, more so to bulbar-related items. Its sensitivity to change or its predictive properties have not been studied.

The Myasthenia Gravis Impairment Index

The Myasthenia Gravis Impairment Index (MGII) has been recently developed using a patient-centered approach, whereby patient input was incorporated through the development process.[12] This method was grounded in a qualitative study of patients' experiences with MG,[9] where fatigability was a key component of overall MG severity. The scale has 22 patient-reported items (2-week recall time) and 6 examination items that reflect severity and fatigability of ocular, bulbar, and limb/generalized impairments. The total scores range between 0 and 84, but it can also be scored as an ocular (0–23) and a generalized (0–61) score, where higher scores indicate greater disease severity. The MGII was validated in a cohort of 200 MG patients.[12] Test–retest reliability for the whole scale and interobserver reliability for the examination component was high (ICCs of 0.93 and 0.90, respectively). Construct validity was tested through predefined hypotheses of the correlations between the MGII and other MG symptoms measures (QMGS, MGC, MG-ADL), an MG-specific HRQoL measure (MG-QoL15), and generic measures (Short Form-36 [SF-36],[42] the EQ-5D,[43] and the NeuroQoL-Fatigue module[44]). Additionally, MGII scores were significantly different across MGFA classes and between ocular/generalized patients, indicating gross discriminative validity.[12] Responsiveness was studied in 95 patients receiving prednisone or immunomodulation (IVIG or plasma exchange), using stable patients from the reliability study as controls.[45] Patients receiving prednisone or immunomodulation changed significantly more than controls. Additionally, patients in the pure ocular group changed significantly in the ocular subscore, without change in generalized items. Overall, patients receiving prednisone changed more in the ocular subscore than those receiving immunomodulation, who changed more in the generalized subscore. Patient-meaningful change was studied using the patient's impression of change, whereby patients who felt better changed significantly more than those who were unchanged or worse. The MID at a group level—to estimate sample size for a trial—was 8.1 points, and at the individual level—to classify a patient as responder—was 5.5 points. The MGII takes approximately 10 minutes to complete, which is feasible depending on the setting. It has not yet been used in a clinical trial.

Special considerations should be made regarding outcomes in patients in myasthenic crisis. Most of these outcomes have been validated in outpatients, so data on crisis are scarce. Many of the physician-rated scales can be applied to patients in crisis, because they usually include intubation/ventilation within the respiratory items. However, patient-reported outcomes by their nature are not suited for these patients, at least in the acute phase.[46] Considering the mortality associated with myasthenic crisis, survival should be a main outcome. Additionally, because MG crisis is defined by the need for intubation, then successful extubation and overall time to extubation have been used to describe the outcomes in this population, because they are associated with the duration of intensive care and hospital stay, medical complications, and overall mortality.[47]

MEASURES OF DISABILITY AND HEALTH-RELATED QUALITY OF LIFE IN MYASTHENIA GRAVIS

There is one measure specifically aimed at measuring disability in MG using the ICF framework, the MG-DIS. Additionally, there are 2 disease-specific measures of HRQoL: the MG-QOL 60, a 60-item measure, and the MG-QOL 15, which derives from the 60 item questionnaire and that has been recently modified (MG-QOL15r). **Table 2** summarizes these measures.

The Myasthenia Gravis Disability Scale

This is a measure specifically developed to quantify disability in patients with MG. The MG-DIS was developed as a patient-reported outcome, using the ICF framework of disability.[48] For this, the authors linked items from available measures to different ICF codes, using previous studies where patients had self-reported their MG-related problems using this classification system.[49] Additionally, the authors conducted semistructured interviews in a group of MG patients, whereby the different codes previously identified where explored in depth, to determine if those symptoms or limitations in activities or participation were directly related to MG. These steps resulted in retaining 42 ICF categories, with a total of 44 preliminary items covering body functions, activities/participation, and environmental factors.[48] The 31 items reflecting impairments and restrictions of activities and participation were further studied for validation.[50] Item reduction was based on interitem correlations and factor analysis, in a cohort of 109 patients, and 20 items were retained.

Table 2
Measures of disability and HRQoL in myasthenia gravis

	Total Items	Score Range	Interpretation
MG-DIS	20	0–100	Higher score, more disability
MG-QOL 60	60	0–240	Higher score, worse HRQoL
MG-QOL 15	15	0–60	Higher score, worse HRQoL
MG- QOL 15 r	15	0–30	Higher score, worse HRQoL

Abbreviations: HRQoL, health-related quality of life; MG-DIS, Myasthenia Gravis Disability Scale; MG-QOL, Myasthenia Gravis Quality of Life.
All these are patient-reported outcomes.

These items reflect generalized impairment problems, bulbar-related problems, mental health and fatigue problems, and vision-related problems. All items have a 30-day recall period, and are graded on a scale of 1 to 5; total scores are transformed to a scale of 0 to 100, where higher scores reflect greater disability. Cronbach's alpha was 0.92, indicating good internal consistency. The test–retest reliability was tested in 21 patients, with high r coefficients. Construct validity was studied through correlations with the MGC as well as fatigability indices, and discriminative validity was tested by comparing MG-DIS scores between ocular/remission patients and patients with generalized disease.[50] Longitudinal data were available for 75 patients, and MG-DIS scores changed according to the patients' impression of change. However, there are no data on the MID and no other studies on responsiveness in relationship to specific interventions.

The Myasthenia Gravis Quality of Life 60

Before this measure was developed, all studies on HRQoL for MG patients used generic measures, such as the SF-36.[42] The aim of the developers was to obtain a measure that would also include the specific effects of MG in HRQoL. Item development was based in a Multiple Sclerosis HRQoL instrument, were experts selected items that were relevant for MG patients.[51] Patients' interviews were conducted and 100 preliminary items were obtained, including physical, social, emotional, and functional problems. The authors obtained feedback from physicians and patients to further reduced the measure to 60 items—each scored in a Likert scale from 0 to 4—resulting in a total score ranging from 0 to 240; higher scores indicate worse HRQoL. The 60-item measure was tested in 80 patients participating in a clinical trial of mycophenolate.[39] Internal consistency was excellent (Cronbach's alpha, 0.94), test–retest reliability was not assessed, given that patients were actively receiving interventions. Construct validity was studied through correlations between the MG-QOL60 and the SF-36 (r = -8.0), the MG-ADL (r = 0.72), the QMGS (r = 0.53), and the MMT (r = 0.43).[51] The MG-QOL60 was used as a secondary outcome in a randomized, controlled study comparing IVIG and plasma exchange.[52] In this study, the MG-QOL60 scores significantly improved in patients receiving both treatments, changing more in responders—who improved by 22 points—compared with those who were unchanged—who changed only by 7 points.[53] However, the MID was not specifically studied.

The Myasthenia Gravis Quality of Life 15 and the Myasthenia Gravis Quality of Life 15 r

The MG-QOL15 was developed with the aim of simplifying the MG-QOL60. First, 20 candidate items were flagged for retention, based on their responsiveness to change in the mycophenolate study.[35] Additionally, data on 13 patients followed in routine clinical visits who reported worsening was assessed, and based on this input the items were reduced to 15: mobility (9 items), symptoms (3 items), and contentment and emotional well-being (3 items). Items are scored in a Likert scale from 0 to 4 and the total sum score ranges from 0 to 60, where higher scores indicate worse HRQoL.[35] The MG-QOL15 has good internal consistency (Cronbach's alpha, 0.89). In terms of construct validity, the MG-QOL15 correlated with the physical and mental components of the SF-36, as well as with MG-specific measures (QMGS, MG-ADL, and MMT).[35] Longitudinal validity was studied in 138 patients with routine follow-up at different centers. Patients were considered improved if they had a 3 or greater point improvement in the MGC and the MG-QOL changed more in those improved compared with those not improved, and the change in QOL-15 scores correlated with the change in MGC (r = 0.53).[54] In the same study, test–retest reliability was excellent (ICC, 0.98). The MG-QOL15 also demonstrated to be responsive in a randomized, controlled study of IVIG versus plasma exchange, where responders to treatment improved in average by 9 points compared with nonresponders, who changed by 2 points, thereby suggesting that a decrease MG QOL-15 of 7 or more points is correlated with improvement in the subgroup with moderate to severe MG (QMGS ≥11).[53] The MID has not been fully determined. The MG-QOL15 has been translated and validated in several languages, such as Japanese and French,[55,56] and it is widely used around the world. Based on its extensive use, it has been recently modified, to improve the performance of certain items.[57] The modified version (MG-QOL15r) retained the 15 items with some wording changes, and these were rescored from a 0 to 4 to a 0 to 2 scale, based on Rasch analysis. The resulting measure scores ranges from 0 to 30, and higher scores indicate worse HRQoL. When compared with the original scale, the modified version had better psychometric properties than the original and it is very easy to use.[57] Responsiveness of the MG-QOLr has not yet been studied.

STEROID-SPARING EFFECTS AND OTHER OUTCOMES

Beyond the symptoms and their effect on the patients' lives, other outcomes have been incorporated in clinical trials of MG, often as biomarkers or surrogate outcomes. Because of the side effects of long-term steroid treatment, it is of interest to measure the overall exposure of prednisone as an outcome, whereby a treatment is superior if it can reduce the use of prednisone over time with good symptomatic control. This steroid-sparing effect has been usually studied using the area under the curve of prednisone over time, for example, in the thymectomy randomized, controlled trial,[36] where the prednisone dose was time weighted and the treated group had a lower prednisone exposure over time than the control arm. Recently, the results of the methotrexate for MG study were published. In this 12-month study, the prednisone area under the curve between months 3 and 12 was the primary outcome.[58] There was no difference in the prednisone area under the curve between the methotrexate and placebo groups; however, more subjects in the placebo arm withdrew from the study and all patients that withdrew owing to worsening MG had received placebo. Finally, some of the secondary measures showed a trend favoring methotrexate. More studies are needed to better understand what difference in overall prednisone exposure is clinically significant. Recently, a study of rituximab on musculoskeletal MG used a composed outcome mixing the MGFA postintervention status and the dose of immunosuppressants, called the Myasthenia Gravis Status and Treatment Intensity Score.[59] Further studies are needed to validate this measure. For more details, the reader is referred to the article by Michael K. Hehir and Nicholas J. Silvestri's article, "Generalized Myasthenia Gravis: Classification, Clinical Presentation, Natural History, and Epidemiology," in this issue.

Electrophysiology testing, such as repetitive nerve stimulation and single fiber electromyography have also been used as surrogate markers of improvement.[60] However, although the decrement on repetitive nerve stimulation and jitter can improve with treatment, their correlation with clinical change is only mild to moderate.[22] Because these tests can be painful and time consuming, they are not routinely used in the follow-up of patients with MG. The titers of acetylcholine receptor antibodies have also been used as biomarker; however, they do not correlate well with clinical change.[61]

SUMMARY

There are several outcome measures available for MG and there is no single, perfect measure that works for every scenario. Because standards for outcome measure development have changed in recent years,[6,7] newer outcomes tend to incorporate more of the patients' input and have more studies on their psychometric properties. Things to take into account when choosing a measure are what it measures, in which population it was validated, what purpose(s) does it serve, and what measurement properties it has. Additionally, feasibility has to be considered—for a busy clinical setting shorter measures might be preferable—whereas in a clinical trial more comprehensive measures might be needed to demonstrate treatment benefits. The validation of measures is an ongoing process, so current measures should be studied in different populations and their responsiveness to different interventions tested.

Finally, more information is needed regarding the interpretation of change scores, to understand what magnitude of change is meaningful. The MIDs should be studied in different settings (ie, groups vs individuals), in patient who are worsening—whose MID is often different than from improvement—and based on baseline severity.[5] Additionally, research into Patient Acceptable Symptom States is needed, aiming to find thresholds for different outcomes were patients are not only a "little better" but "good enough."[62] These Patient Acceptable Symptom States thresholds could eventually serve as therapeutic targets both for clinical and research settings.

REFERENCES

1. Jette AM. Toward a common language for function, disability, and health. Phys Ther 2006;86(5):726–34.
2. World Health Organization. International classification of functioning, disability and health (ICF). 1st edition. Geneva: World Health Organization; 2002. Available at: http://www.who.int/classifications/icf/icfbeginnersguide.pdf?ua=1. Accessed June, 2017.
3. Guyatt GH, Bombardier C, Tugwell PX. Measuring disease-specific quality of life in clinical trials. Can Med Assoc J 1986;134:889.
4. Kirshner B, Guyatt G. A methodological framework for assessing health indices. J Chronic Dis 1985;38(1):27–36.
5. King MT. A point of minimal important difference (MID): a critique of terminology and methods. Expert Rev Pharmacoecon Outcomes Res 2011;11(2):171–84.
6. U.S. Department of Health and Human Services FDA Center for Drug Evaluation and Research, U.S. Department of Health and Human Services FDA Center for Biologics Evaluation and Research, U.S. Department of Health and Human Services FDA Center for Devices and Radiological Health. Guidance for industry: patient-reported outcome measures: use in medical product development to support labeling claims: draft guidance. Health Qual Life Outcomes 2006;4:79.
7. Mokkink LB, Terwee CB, Knol DL, et al. The COSMIN checklist for evaluating the methodological quality of studies on measurement properties: a clarification of its content. BMC Med Res Methodol 2010;10(1):22.
8. De Vet HCW, Terwee CB, Mokkink LB, et al. Measurement in medicine. New York: Cambridge University Press; 2011.
9. Barnett C, Bril V, Kapral M, et al. A conceptual framework for evaluating impairments in myasthenia gravis. PLoS One 2014;9(5):e98089.
10. Wolfe GI, Herbelin L, Nations SP, et al. Myasthenia gravis activities of daily living profile. Neurology 1999;52(7):1487–9.

11. Burns TM, Conaway MR, Cutter GR, et al, Muscle Study Group. Construction of an efficient evaluative instrument for myasthenia gravis: the MG composite. Muscle Nerve 2008;38(6):1553–62.

12. Barnett C, Bril V, Kapral M, et al. Development and validation of the myasthenia gravis impairment index. Neurology 2016;87(9):879–86.

13. Osserman KE, Kornfeld P, Cohen E, et al. Studies in myasthenia gravis; review of two hundred eighty-two cases at the Mount Sinai Hospital, New York City. AMA Arch Intern Med 1958;102(1):72–81.

14. Jaretzki A, Barohn RJ, Ernstoff RM, et al. Myasthenia gravis: recommendations for clinical research standards. Task Force of the Medical Scientific Advisory Board of the Myasthenia Gravis Foundation of America. Neurology 2000;55(1): 16–23.

15. Baggi F, Mantegazza R, Antozzi C, et al. Patient registries: useful tools for clinical research in myasthenia gravis. Ann N Y Acad Sci 2012;1274(1):107–13.

16. Besinger UA, Toyka KV, Homberg M, et al. Myasthenia gravis: long-term correlation of binding and bungarotoxin blocking antibodies against acetylcholine receptors with changes in disease severity. Neurology 1983;33(10):1316–21.

17. Tindall RS, Rollins JA, Phillips JT, et al. Preliminary results of a double-blind, randomized, placebo-controlled trial of cyclosporine in myasthenia gravis. N Engl J Med 1987;316(12):719–24.

18. Barohn RJ, McIntire D, Herbelin L, et al. Reliability testing of the quantitative myasthenia gravis score. Ann N Y Acad Sci 1998;841:769–72.

19. Sharshar T, Chevret S, Mazighi M, et al. Validity and reliability of two muscle strength scores commonly used as endpoints in assessing treatment of myasthenia gravis. J Neurol 2000;247(4):286–90.

20. Barnett C, Merkies ISJ, Katzberg H, et al. Psychometric properties of the quantitative myasthenia gravis score and the myasthenia gravis composite scale. J Neuromuscul Dis 2015;2(3):301–11.

21. Sanders DB, Tucker-Lipscomb B, Massey J. A simple manual muscle test for myasthenia gravis: validation and comparison with the QMG score. Ann N Y Acad Sci 2003;998:440–4.

22. Barnett C, Katzberg H, Navabi M, et al. The quantitative myasthenia gravis score: comparison with clinical, electrophysiological, and laboratory markers. J Clin Neuromuscul Dis 2012;13(4):201–5.

23. Bedlack RS, Simel DL, Bosworth H, et al. Quantitative myasthenia gravis score: assessment of responsiveness and longitudinal validity. Neurology 2005;64(11): 1968–70.

24. Zinman L, Ng E, Bril V. IV immunoglobulin in patients with myasthenia gravis: a randomized controlled trial. Neurology 2007;68(11):837–41.

25. Katzberg HD, Barnett C, Merkies ISJ, et al. Minimal clinically important difference in myasthenia gravis: outcomes from a randomized trial. Muscle Nerve 2014; 49(5):661–5.

26. Barnett TC, Bril V, Davis AM. Performance of individual items of the quantitative myasthenia gravis score. Neuromuscul Disord 2013;23(5):413–7.

27. Gajdos P, Simon N, de Rohan-Chabot P, et al. Long-term effects of plasma exchange in myasthenia. Results of a randomized study. Presse Med 1983; 12(15):939–42 [in French].

28. Gajdos P, Chevret S, Clair B, et al. Clinical trial of plasma exchange and high-dose intravenous immunoglobulin in myasthenia gravis. Myasthenia Gravis Clinical Study Group. Ann Neurol 1997;41(6):789–96.

29. Mantegazza R, Antozzi C, Peluchetti D. Azathioprine as a single drug or in combination with steroids in the treatment of myasthenia gravis. J Neurol 1988;235: 449–53.

30. Antozzi C, Brenna G, Baggi F, et al. Validation of the Besta Neurological Institute Rating Scale for Myasthenia Gravis. Muscle Nerve 2015;53(1):32–7.

31. Lashley D, Palace J, Jayawant S, et al. Ephedrine treatment in congenital myasthenic syndrome due to mutations in DOK7. Neurology 2010;74(19):1517–23.

32. Wolfe GI, Barohn RJ, Foster BM, et al. Randomized, controlled trial of intravenous immunoglobulin in myasthenia gravis. Muscle Nerve 2002;26(4):549–52.

33. Muppidi S, Wolfe GI, Conaway M, Burns T and the MG Composite and MG-QOL15 Study Group. MG-ADL: still a relevant outcome measure. Muscle Nerve 2011;44(5):727–31.

34. Burns TM, Conaway M, Sanders DB, MG Composite and MG-QOL15 Study Group. The MG composite: a valid and reliable outcome measure for myasthenia gravis. Neurology 2010;74(18):1434–40.

35. Burns TB, Conaway MR, Cutter GR, et al, The Muscle Study Group. Less is more, or almost as much: a 15-item quality-of-life instrument for myasthenia gravis. Muscle Nerve 2008;38(2):957–63.

36. Wolfe GI, Kaminski HJ, Aban IB, et al. Randomized trial of thymectomy in myasthenia gravis. N Engl J Med 2016;375(6):511–22.

37. Sanders DB, Hart IK, Mantegazza R, et al. An international, phase III, randomized trial of mycophenolate mofetil in myasthenia gravis. Neurology 2008;71(6):400–6.

38. Wolfe GI, Barohn RJ, Sanders DB, et al. Comparison of outcome measures from a trial of Mycophenolate mofetil in myasthenia gravis. Muscle Nerve 2008;38(5):1429–33.

39. Muscle Study Group. A trial of mycophenolate mofetil with prednisone as initial immunotherapy in myasthenia gravis. Neurology 2008;71(6):394–9.

40. Benatar M, Sanders DB, Burns TM, et al. Recommendations for myasthenia gravis clinical trials. Muscle Nerve 2012;45:909–17.

41. Farrugia ME, Harle HD, Carmichael C, et al. The oculobulbar facial respiratory score is a tool to assess bulbar function in myasthenia gravis patients. Muscle Nerve 2011;43(3):329–34.

42. Ware JE, Snow KK, Kosinski M, et al. SF-36 health survey. Boston: Manual and Interpretation Guide. New England Medical Center Hospital. Health Institute; 1993.

43. Rabin R, de Charro F. EQ-5D: a measure of health status from the EuroQol Group. Ann Med 2001;33(5):337–43.

44. Cook KF, Victorson DE, Cella D, et al. Creating meaningful cut-scores for Neuro-QOL measures of fatigue, physical functioning, and sleep disturbance using standard setting with patients and providers. Qual Life Res 2014;24(3):575–89.

45. Barnett C, Vera B, Kapral M, et al. Myasthenia Gravis Impairment Index: Responsiveness, meaningful change, and relative efficiency. Neurology 2017;89(23):2357–64.

46. Heyland DK, Guyatt G, Cook DJ, et al. Frequency and methodologic rigor of quality-of-life assessments in the critical care literature. Crit Care Med 1998; 26(3):591–8.

47. Ramos-Fransi A, Rojas-García R, Segovia S, et al. Myasthenia gravis: descriptive analysis of life-threatening events in a recent nationwide registry. Eur J Neurol 2015;22(7):1056–61.

48. Raggi A, Schiavolin S, Leonardi M, et al. Development of the MG-DIS: an ICF-based disability assessment instrument for myasthenia gravis. Disabil Rehabil 2014;36(7):546–55.

49. Leonardi M, Raggi A, Antozzi C, et al. Identification of international classification of functioning, disability and health relevant categories to describe functioning

and disability of patients with myasthenia gravis. Disabil Rehabil 2009;31(24): 2041–6.

50. Raggi A, Leonardi M, Schiavolin S, et al. Validation of the MG-DIS: a disability assessment for myasthenia gravis. J Neurol 2016;263(5):871–82.

51. Mullins LL, Carpentier MY, Paul RH, Sanders DB and the Muscle Study Group. Disease-specific measure of quality of life for myasthenia gravis. Muscle Nerve 2008;38(2):947–56.

52. Barth D, Nabavi Nouri M, Ng E, et al. Comparison of IVIg and PLEX in patients with myasthenia gravis. Neurology 2011;76(23):2017–23.

53. Barnett C, Wilson G, Barth D, et al. Changes in quality of life scores with intravenous immunoglobulin or plasmapheresis in patients with myasthenia gravis. J Neurol Neurosurg Psychiatry 2013;84(1):94–7.

54. Burns TM, Grouse CK, Wolfe GI, et al. The MG-QOL15 for following the health-related quality of life of patients with myasthenia gravis. Muscle Nerve 2011; 43(1):14–8.

55. Masuda M, Utsugisawa K, Suzuki S, et al. The MG-QOL15 Japanese version: validation and associations with clinical factors. Muscle Nerve 2012;46(2): 166–73.

56. Birnbaum S, Ghout I, Demeret S, et al. Translation, cross-cultural adaptation, and validation of the French version of the 15-item myasthenia gravis quality of life scale. Muscle Nerve 2017;55(5):639–45.

57. Burns TM, Sadjadi R, Utsugisawa K, et al. An international clinimetric evaluation of the MG-QOL15, resulting in slight revision and subsequent validation of the MG-QOL15r. Muscle Nerve 2016;54(6):1015–22.

58. Pasnoor M, He J, Herbelin L, et al. A randomized controlled trial of methotrexate for patients with generalized myasthenia gravis. Neurology 2016;87(1):57–64.

59. Hehir M, Hobson-Webb LD, Benatar M, et al. Rituximab as treatment for anti-MuSK myasthenia gravis: multicenter blinded prospective review. Neurology 2017;89(10):1069–77.

60. Zinman L, Baryshnik D, Bril V. Surrogate therapeutic outcome measures in patients with myasthenia gravis. Muscle Nerve 2008;37(2):172–6.

61. Sanders DB, Burns TM, Cutter GR, et al. Does change in acetylcholine receptor antibody level correlate with clinical change in myasthenia gravis? Muscle Nerve 2014;49(4):483–6.

62. Wijeysundera DN, Johnson SR. How much better is good enough? Patient-reported outcomes, minimal clinically important differences, and patient acceptable symptom states in perioperative research. Anesthesiology 2016;125(1): 7–10.

An Update
Myasthenia Gravis and Pregnancy

Johanna Hamel, MD[a],*, Emma Ciafaloni, MD[b]

KEYWORDS

- Pregnancy • Myasthenia gravis • Neonatal myasthenia gravis • Arthrogryposis

KEY POINTS

- Women with myasthenia gravis considering pregnancy should meet with their neurologist to review the role of thymectomy, maximize clinical improvement, and minimize the use of immunomodulating medications before conception.
- Treatment goal is minimal disease activity in the mother with minimal risk for harm to the fetus.
- The treatment team should include the neurologist, the obstetrician, and the anesthesiologist to support the patient during pregnancy and postpartum period, and to plan optimal mode of delivery.
- Newborns of mothers with myasthenia are at risk of transient neonatal myasthenia gravis and should be monitored for symptoms of myasthenia.
- Pregnancy outcome is generally favorable in women with myasthenia gravis who receive treatment.

INTRODUCTION: CONCEPTS OF TREATING WOMEN WITH MYASTHENIA GRAVIS IN THE CHILDBEARING AGE AND DURING PREGNANCY

Although myasthenia gravis (MG) can affect men and women at any age, female incidence peaks in the second and third decade, and therefore coincides with family planning and fertility. The first step when establishing care with a patient with MG is to confirm the diagnosis, either by detecting antibodies against the nicotinic acetylcholine receptor (AchR-Ab) or other postsynaptic antigens, such as muscle-specific tyrosine kinase (MuSK-Ab) and low-density lipoprotein receptor-related protein 4. In seronegative patients repetitive nerve stimulation testing or single-fiber electromyography is diagnostic by confirming dysfunction of the neuromuscular junction. Issues related to the

Disclosure Statement: The authors have nothing to disclose.
a Department of Neurology, Neuromuscular Division, University of Rochester Medical Center, University of Rochester, 601 Elmwood Avenue, Rochester, NY 14642, USA; b University of Rochester Medical Center, University of Rochester, 601 Elmwood Avenue, PO Box 673, Rochester, NY 14642, USA
* Corresponding author.
E-mail address: Johanna_hamel@urmc.rochester.edu

care of patients with MG in the childbearing age may include questions about fertility, pregnancy planning, drug safety, and treatment optimization preceding conception. Disease severity varies between patients but also within an individual over time. Symptoms can vary throughout pregnancy, thus patients need to be aware of how to monitor and react to changes in their symptoms because treatment adjustments may become necessary. An individualized treatment plan is important, taking into account the patient's disease manifestations, comorbidities, and treatment goals. The pregnancy can affect the course of myasthenia, and the myasthenia can affect the pregnancy outcome and cause transient neonatal myasthenia and in rare circumstances arthrogryposis in the newborn. Although myasthenia does not affect smooth muscle, labor and delivery relies on striated muscle in the later stages, which can be prolonged. Certain medications, such as anesthetics, can worsen symptoms of MG. Lastly, symptoms can vary in puerperium and drug safety during lactation needs to be discussed.

TREATMENT AND DRUG SAFETY BEFORE PREGNANCY

Although MG itself does not affect fertility, immunosuppressive medications commonly used in MG do. Conversations between a woman with MG and her neurologist about fertility and pregnancy planning should begin early, such as when choosing an immunosuppressive therapy. Methotrexate (MTX) and mycophenolate mofetil (MMF) are contraindicated in women who try to conceive and should be discontinued 3 months (MTX) and 6 weeks (MMF) before conception.[1] Azathioprine and corticosteroids are continued because they do not seem to affect fertility.[2] Women treated with rituximab (RTX) are advised to use contraception 12 months after the last treatment. Effects of RTX on fertility beyond the 12-month period are not well known. However, a case series described two uncomplicated pregnancies in two patients previously treated with RTX.[3] Thymectomy improves clinical outcomes, reduces use of immunosuppressive agents, and is recommended for patients younger than age 65.[4] If a patient is planning to become pregnant, but has not yet had thymectomy, it should be considered to optimize disease control.[5] Patients who had undergone thymectomy seemed to have a lower likelihood of neonatal myasthenia in the infant.[6,7] However, thymectomy did not affect severity of symptoms, use of medication, and complications with delivery.[7]

TREATMENT AND DRUG SAFETY DURING PREGNANCY

Ideally a patient and the treating neurologist discuss treatment goals and options before becoming pregnant. Optimizing treatment before and during pregnancy with best possible safety profile for the patient and the fetus is of key importance. Depending on the patient's duration and type of symptoms (eg, ocular vs bulbar) and symptom severity, discontinuation of immunosuppressive therapy might be considered before conception. However, if a patient is already pregnant, discontinuation of therapy with the risk of worsening of myasthenic symptoms or of triggering myasthenic crisis often outweighs the risk of the unwanted medication effects on the fetus. Most recommendations related to drug safety are based on retrospective analysis, observational or animal studies, or stem from experiences with immunosuppressive medications when used in other diseases.

Treatment of MG includes symptomatic and immunosuppressive/immunomodulatory treatment. Treatment of choice during pregnancy is pyridostigmine and corticosteroids. It is not recommend starting other immunosuppressive agents because the effect of treatment can be delayed by many months and would not benefit the disease course during pregnancy itself, while increasing the risk of possible harm to the infant. If a patient is already on azathioprine or cyclo-sporine, it is considered safe to continue these medications throughout pregnancy. For acute exacerbation of MG or myasthenic crisis, intravenous immunoglobulin (IVIG) can be used safely if needed and possibly plasmapheresis, although the latter may remove hormones important to maintenance of the fetus. Hyperemesis gravidarum may complicate therapy because of limited absorption of the medications and should be assessed as a possible (treatable) cause in case of an exacerbation. **Table 1** summarizes treatment recommendations and drug safety.

Treatment of Choice

Pyridostigmine
Symptomatic treatment with pyridostigmine can provide sufficient symptom control for patients with mild disease manifestations or isolated ocular symptoms. Doses

Table 1			
Treatment recommendations and drug safety for patients with MG prior, during, and after pregnancy			
Medication/ Intervention	**Preconception**	**Pregnancy**	**Lactation**
Treatment of choice			
Pyridostigmine	No limitations	<600 mg/d	Larger doses can cause gastrointestinal discomfort in the fetus
Corticosteroids	No limitations	lowest effective dose	No limitations
Treatment of choice for exacerbation of MG crisis			
IVIG	No limitations	Treatment of choice	No limitations
Plasma exchange	No limitations	Monitor fluid shifts	No limitations
Treatment considered for continuation (but not initiation during)			
Cyclosporine	Contraception recommended	Continuation of therapy can be considered if needed	Can be considered
Azathioprine	Contraception recommended	Continuation of therapy can be considered if needed	Considered acceptable not by all but most experts
Contraindicated/discontinuation recommended			
Methotrexate	Strict contraception recommended until 3 mo after discontinuation	Contraindicated	Contraindicated
Mycophenolate mofetil	Contraception recommended until 6 wk after discontinuation	Discontinuation recommended	Not recommended because of lack of information
Unknown risks			
Rituximab	Not recommended because of lack of information	Not recommended because of lack of information	Not recommended because of lack of information

less than 600 mg/day are safe for the fetus. Intravenous cholinesterase inhibitors should be avoided during pregnancy because of the risk of uterine contractions.[8]

Corticosteroids
Patients not in remission or with insufficient symptom control on pyridostigmine require immunosuppressive therapy. Corticosteroids (prednisone) is the treatment of choice given its low teratogenic risk to the fetus with only a slight increased risk of cleft palate when used in the first trimester.[9] Higher doses of corticosteroids have been associated with premature rupture of the membranes and gestational diabetes.[1]

Immunoglobulins
IVIG is used to control symptoms of MG that do not respond to corticosteroids or pyridostigmine, and to manage myasthenic crisis in pregnancy. The safety of IVIG in pregnancy has not been investigated in MG itself but has been well documented in other disorders including neurologic autoimmune conditions, such as multiple sclerosis.[10] Side effects, such as hyperviscosity and volume overload, may be more relevant in pregnancy.

Plasmapheresis
Theoretically, plasmapheresis may induce premature delivery because of large hormonal shifts.[11] Variations of the oncotic pressure may cause fluctuations in blood pressure that are able to interfere with the flow of placental blood. Removal of coagulation factors and IgG may result in increased risk of bleeding and infection. However, despite these theoretic concerns, plasmapheresis has been used successfully in pregnant patients with MG and for other indications.[12]

Treatments to be Considered

Azathioprine
Azathioprine has been shown to be teratogenic in animals, but clinical experience in women with organ transplants has been reassuring.[1,13] However, intrauterine growth restriction and preterm delivery have been associated with azathioprine use. The risk of fetal immunosuppression and pancytopenia seem to be lower when the maternal leukocyte counts remain in the reference range.[1]

Cyclosporine
Although no teratogenicity has been demonstrated in humans, intrauterine growth restriction is seen.

Medications that Should Not be Used in Pregnancy

Mycophenolate mofetil
MMF has been associated with an increased risk of first trimester miscarriage and increased number of congenital malformations especially cleft lip, and malformations of ears, palate, distal limbs, esophagus, kidney, and central nervous system.

Methotrexate
MTX has been shown to be teratogenic and associated with an increased rate of miscarriages.[1,13]

Rituximab
There are limited data on the safe use of RTX in pregnancy and this medication should be replaced by alternate therapy before conception. A case series reported successful

healthy pregnancies in patients with prior treatment with RTX, which was completed greater than 12 months before conception.[3,13]

TREATMENT AND DRUG SAFETY AFTER PREGNANCY (LACTATION)

Available information on drug safety is mostly based on experiences with patients with organ transplants. A maternal dose of corticosteroids of less than 20 mg/day in a breastfeeding mother results in low levels of the drug in breast milk and is not associated with negative side effects on the newborn.[14] Breastfeeding while taking azathioprine or cyclosporine is considered safe with no adverse effects on exposed children.[14] Some authors suggest to avoid breastfeeding close to peak serum concentration.[1] Breastfeeding safety of MMF is uncertain. The body of data will likely not expand in the future because patients planning to conceive or pregnant should discontinue MMF and likely will stay off the medication postpartum, because initiation of the drug would not provide immediate benefit. Breast feeding safety of RTX is uncertain and therefore should be avoided.[13]

PREGNANCY
Influence of the Pregnancy on Myasthenia Gravis

- The long-term outcome of MG is not affected by pregnancy.[11]
- Pregnancy and eventually parenthood imposes additional physical challenges to a woman with MG. A commitment to more frequent monitoring and increased treatment might become necessary.
- Anticipating the disease course of MG during pregnancy is limited because it is highly variable and unpredictable, independent of severity of symptoms before conception or experiences with previous pregnancies. A recent study suggested that duration of MG, MG composite score, and repetitive nerve stimulation before pregnancy may be useful in helping to predict the course of MG during pregnancy,[15] although these findings warrant replication.
- One-third of women experience worsening of symptoms, mostly in the first trimester or postpartum.[11,16] One study from Brazil reported exacerbation of MG in a higher percentage (50%) of patients, mostly in the second trimester.[15]
  - Improvement in symptoms or even complete remission is seen in the second or third trimester, thought to be related to the physiologic immunosuppression induced by high level of α-fetoprotein (AFP) that occurs during those phases of gestation.[6,15–17] This may also explain exacerbations postpartum, as the AFP levels fall.
- Attention should be given to changes in respiratory function because the enlarging uterus may restrict the diaphragm.[16] A baseline forced vital capacity should be obtained and repeated as needed with any changes throughout pregnancy.
- Triggers for myasthenic crisis or MG exacerbations in general, but also in pregnancy, include infections,[15] which are more common during pregnancy because of changes in the immune system. Infections should be treated without delay. Caution is warranted with use of antibiotics that have the potential to trigger myasthenic crisis (eg, fluoroquinolones, aminoglycosides).

Myasthenia Gravis as a New Diagnosis During Pregnancy or Postpartum

Women can develop their first symptoms of MG during pregnancy or postpartum. Changes in the immune system, such as estrogen-induced cytokine or immunoglobulin production, and a drop of AFP following delivery, along with stress and sleep deprivation are all possible triggers. In a cross-sectional case-controlled study from Norway, pregnancy preceded the onset of MG in 15%. The relative risk to develop MG in the postpartum period, specifically the first 3 months after birth of the first child, was significantly increased (relative risk, 5.5).[18] In another study 12% of mothers with MG developed their first symptoms or were diagnosed during their first pregnancy.[7] In rare circumstances, the patient can present with myasthenic crisis as the first symptom during pregnancy.[19]

Diagnostic work-up for a new diagnosis of MG during pregnancy includes the following:

- AChR-Ab testing. If negative, test for anti- MuSK and lipoprotein receptor-related protein 4.
- If antibody negative, repetitive nerve stimulation or single-fiber electromyogram to confirm dysfunction of the neuromuscular junction (safe during pregnancy).
- Chest imaging to look for thymoma should be postponed until after the delivery: there is no indication for thymectomy during pregnancy because of its delayed effect, no benefit would be expected from the intervention during pregnancy.[8] In addition, most thymomas are benign and slow growing and urgent removal is not necessary.

Influence of Myasthenia Gravis on the Pregnancy and the Fetus

In a Taiwanese study with 163 patients, there was no statistically significant increased risk of preterm birth, low birth weight, or infants small for gestational age.[20] Women with MG have no increased risk of spontaneous abortion.[7]

Delivery and postpartum

Although MG does not result in an increased risk for complications during the course of a pregnancy, there is an increased risk for complications and a need for interventions during delivery (affecting up to 30% of patients).[7,21] **Table 2** provides an overview of available studies and reported complications. All listed studies were carried out with retrospective design except one (Batocchi and colleagues[11]). The mother's clinical status does not predict complications during delivery, which is seen even in asymptomatic patients.[22] Most common complications include protracted labor and fetal distress.[7,21] Because the second phase of delivery relies on voluntary pushing efforts of the mother, which involves striated muscles, fatigue can occur. Use of forceps or vacuum extraction can help to ease the second labor stage.[6] In addition, parenteral anticholinesterase medications can help strengthen the muscle, because oral absorption is limited. Caution is warranted with transitioning from oral to intravenous dosing: a dose of 60 mg oral pyridostigmine is equivalent to 2 mg of pyridostigmine intravenously, 1.5 mg neostigmine intramuscularly, or 0.5 mg neostigmine intravenously. MG itself is not an indication for C-section[6] and C-section should only be performed for standard obstetric indications or severe exacerbations. Emergent C-sections typically involve general anesthesia and should be avoided if possible, because patients with MG are sensitive to anesthetic agents. Anesthesia considerations are as follows:

- Medications to avoid in labor because they can result in worsening of weakness:
  - Nondepolarizing muscle relaxants
  - Magnesium: barbiturates or phenytoin are considered alternate therapies for eclampsia instead[8]

Table 2
Complications during pregnancy

Study	No. Pregnancies/ Patients	Treatment	Disease Course Pregnancy/ Postpartum	C-Section	Vaginal Intervention (Vacuum/ Forceps)	Protracted Labor	Preterm Rupture of Membranes	Other Findings
Ducci et al,[15] 2017 Brazil	35/21	Third trimester maintenance: pyridostigmine, 28; CS, 19; azathioprine, 2	50% worsened (mainly during the second trimester), 30% improved, 20% no change	66.7%[a] (15 with obstetric indication and 5 caused by worsening of MG)	6.7%	NA	25.8%	Worsening group more likely to have abnormal RNS[b] and lower MGC scores[b] before pregnancy Improvement group: higher MGC scores[b] before pregnancy No-change group: longer disease duration of MG[b] and normal RNS[b] before pregnancy
Almeida et al,[19] 2010 Portugal	17/17 (2 abortions)	At partum: 8 on CS, 5 on IVIG, 9 on pyridostigmine, 4 untreated (3 new diagnoses, 1 in remission)	8 no change, 4 with worsening, 3 mild symptoms (first manifestation)/3 with MG crisis postpartal (2 untreated with new diagnosis)	Nonurgent in 8/ 17 (7 from obstetric causes)	NA	NA	13.3%	4 with spinal block, 10 with epidural block or analgesia, 13/15 pregnancies full term

(continued on next page)

Table 2
(continued)

Study	No. Pregnancies/ Patients	Treatment	Disease Course Pregnancy/ Postpartum	C-Section	Vaginal Intervention (Vacuum/ Forceps)[a]	Protracted Labor	Preterm Rupture of Membranes	Other Findings
Wen et al,[20] 2009 Taiwan	163	NA	NA	NS (44.8% but 37.4% in control group)[a]	10.0% (vs 10.2%)	NS	NS	No increased risk of preterm, low birth weight, and small for gestational age infants
Hoff et al,[21] 2003 Norway/ Hoff et al,[7] 2007 Dutch	135/73	Pyridostigmine, 66; CS, 1; plasmapheresis, 3	10% worsened	17.3% (many elective vs 8.6%)[b]	8.7%	19%	5.5% (vs 1.7%)[b]	Patients with mild MG/ remission Risk for neonatal MG was halved if the mother was thymectomized
Djelmis et al,[6] 2002 Croatia	69/65	23.2% not on treatment (remission), 43.5% on pyridostigmine only, 33.3% on pyridostigmine + CS, 9 plasmapheresis	15% deteriorated in pregnancy, 16% in the puerperium	17% (all but one for obstetric reasons)	9%	NA	NA	Shorter disease duration and infection predispose to puerperal exacerbation Maternal thymectomy lessens the likelihood of neonatal myasthenia

| Batocchi et al,[11] 1999 Italy | 64/47 | 30 on pyridostigmine, 7 on CS, 4 on azathioprine, 2 on IVIG and plasmapheresis | Relapse in 17% of asymptomatic patients not on therapy; in patients on therapy, improvement in 39%, unchanged in 42%, worsened in 19% Postpartal worsening in 28% | 30%, most for obstetric reasons | NA | NA | NA | NA | No correlation between MG severity before conception and exacerbation of symptoms during pregnancy No increased prevalence of premature labor or low birth weight |

Note that a high cesarean rate in the general population can mask the possibility of an even higher rate of cesarean delivery among specific risk groups, compared with unaffected women.

Abbreviations: CS, corticosteroids; MGC score, myasthenia gravis composite score; NA, not assessed; NS, not significant; RNS, repetitive nerve stimulation.
[a] Despite these insignificant differences.
[b] Statistically significant (eg, when compared with reference group).

- Epidural analgesia is the preferred anesthetic modality in women with MG: it can prevent or reduce the administration of potentially respiratory depressant systemic analgesics, regulate breathing, and reduce fatigability[19]
- Spinal anesthesia has been safely used for several patients in C-sections[15]

Neonatal myasthenia gravis

Transient neonatal MG (NMG) is a clinical diagnosis in the newborn characterized by self-limited generalized hypotonia and weakness; ptosis; and extraocular, bulbar, and respiratory muscle involvement of variable severity. Symptoms typically occur within 48 hours after birth and last for 1 month but on occasion can occur a few days after and persist from 2 weeks to several months. Monitoring of the newborn for at least 48 hours and counseling of the parents about symptoms to monitor is important.[9] Children with NMG have been associated with higher incidence of distress and hypoxia at birth.[7] The syndrome is caused by transplacental transmission of maternal AchR-Ab and has been described in 10% to 20% of children born to mothers with MG.[6,7,11] More recently several case reports have described NMG in women with anti-MuSK antibodies.[23–25] There is no maternal predictor to anticipate the risk of a newborn to have NMG, because the occurrence does not correlate with maternal disease severity or antibody titers.[6,11] The only association found in some studies is that a history of thymectomy in the mother seems to decrease the risk of NMG.[6,7] Treatment is supportive and depends on symptom severity: for mild symptoms neostigmine is sufficient; for more severe cases with respiratory involvement, plasmapheresis needs to be considered.

Arthrogryposis

Arthrogryposis multiplex congenita is a clinical description of nonprogressive contractures involving more than two joints in a neonate. This syndrome is caused by several conditions, including neuromuscular diseases. In rare instances it can occur in patients with MG, because of placental transmission of antibodies against the fetal AchR resulting in decreased fetal intrauterine movements. Severity is variable and ranges from mild contractures to fetal or neonatal death.[26] Just as in NMG, the mother's disease course or antibody status does not serve as a predictor. However, if a woman already had a child with arthrogryposis, there is a higher risk of recurrence in subsequent pregnancies.[27] Monitoring fetal movements and joint contractures with ultrasound is helpful, although there is no treatment to reverse the process. Although plasmapheresis in the mother may be a theoretic consideration, there are no experience or data to support this.

REFERENCES

1. Durst JK, Rampersad RM. Pregnancy in women with solid-organ transplants: a review. Obstet Gynecol Surv 2015;70(6):408–18.
2. Leroy C, Rigot JM, Leroy M, et al. Immunosuppressive drugs and fertility. Orphanet J Rare Dis 2015;10:136.
3. Stieglbauer K, Pichler R, Topakian R. 10-year-outcomes after rituximab for myasthenia gravis: efficacy, safety, costs of inhospital care, and impact on childbearing potential. J Neurol Sci 2017;375:241–4.
4. Wolfe GI, Kaminski HJ, Sonnett JR, et al. Randomized trial of thymectomy in myasthenia gravis. J Thorac Dis 2016;8(12):E1782–3.
5. Norwood F, Dhanjal M, Hill M, et al. Myasthenia in pregnancy: best practice guidelines from a U.K. multispecialty working group. J Neurol Neurosurg Psychiatry 2014;85(5):538–43.

6. Djelmis J, Sostarko M, Mayer D, et al. Myasthenia gravis in pregnancy: report on 69 cases. Eur J Obstet Gynecol Reprod Biol 2002;104(1):21–5.
7. Hoff JM, Daltveit AK, Gilhus NE. Myasthenia gravis in pregnancy and birth: identifying risk factors, optimising care. Eur J Neurol 2007;14(1):38–43.
8. Sanders DB, Wolfe GI, Benatar M, et al. International consensus guidance for management of myasthenia gravis: executive summary. Neurology 2016;87(4): 419–25.
9. Ciafaloni E, Massey JM. Myasthenia gravis and pregnancy. Neurol Clin 2004; 22(4):771–82.
10. Feasby T, Banwell B, Benstead T, et al. Guidelines on the use of intravenous immune globulin for neurologic conditions. Transfus Med Rev 2007;21(2 Suppl 1): S57–107.
11. Batocchi AP, Majolini L, Evoli A, et al. Course and treatment of myasthenia gravis during pregnancy. Neurology 1999;52(3):447–52.
12. Marson P, Gervasi MT, Tison T, et al. Therapeutic apheresis in pregnancy: general considerations and current practice. Transfus Apher Sci 2015;53(3):256–61.
13. Götestam Skorpen C, Hoeltzenbein M, Tincani A, et al. The EULAR points to consider for use of antirheumatic drugs before pregnancy, and during pregnancy and lactation. Ann Rheum Dis 2016;75(5):795–810.
14. Constantinescu S, Pai A, Coscia LA, et al. Breast-feeding after transplantation. Best Pract Res Clin Obstet Gynaecol 2014;28(8):1163–73.
15. Ducci RD, Lorenzoni PJ, Kay CS, et al. Clinical follow-up of pregnancy in myasthenia gravis patients. Neuromuscul Disord 2017;27(4):352–7.
16. Ciafaloni E, Massey JM. The management of myasthenia gravis in pregnancy. Semin Neurol 2004;24(1):95–100.
17. Ferrero S, Pretta S, Nicoletti A, et al. Myasthenia gravis: management issues during pregnancy. Eur J Obstet Gynecol Reprod Biol 2005;121(2):129–38.
18. Boldingh MI, Maniaol AH, Brunborg C, et al. Increased risk for clinical onset of myasthenia gravis during the postpartum period. Neurology 2016;87(20): 2139–45.
19. Almeida C, Coutinho E, Moreira D, et al. Myasthenia gravis and pregnancy: anaesthetic management–a series of cases. Eur J Anaesthesiol 2010;27(11): 985–90.
20. Wen JC, Liu TC, Chen YH, et al. No increased risk of adverse pregnancy outcomes for women with myasthenia gravis: a nationwide population-based study. Eur J Neurol 2009;16(8):889–94.
21. Hoff JM, Daltveit AK, Gilhus NE. Myasthenia gravis: consequences for pregnancy, delivery, and the newborn. Neurology 2003;61(10):1362–6.
22. Hoff JM, Daltveit AK, Gilhus NE. Asymptomatic myasthenia gravis influences pregnancy and birth. Eur J Neurol 2004;11(8):559–62.
23. Lee JY, Min JH, Han SH, et al. Transient neonatal myasthenia gravis due to a mother with ocular onset of anti-muscle specific kinase myasthenia gravis. Neuromuscul Disord 2017;27(7):655–7.
24. Behin A, Mayer M, Kassis-Makhoul B, et al. Severe neonatal myasthenia due to maternal anti-MuSK antibodies. Neuromuscul Disord 2008;18(6):443–6.
25. Niks EH, Verrips A, Semmekrot BA, et al. A transient neonatal myasthenic syndrome with anti-musk antibodies. Neurology 2008;70(14):1215–6.
26. Vincent A, Newland C, Brueton L, et al. Arthrogryposis multiplex congenita with maternal autoantibodies specific for a fetal antigen. Lancet 1995;346(8966):24–5.
27. Midelfart Hoff J, Midelfart A. Maternal myasthenia gravis: a cause for arthrogryposis multiplex congenita. J Child Orthop 2015;9(6):433–5.

Congenital Myasthenic Syndromes

Perry B. Shieh, MD, PhD[a],*, Shin J. Oh, MD[b]

KEYWORDS

- Congenital myasthenic syndrome • Neuromuscular junction • Safety factor
- Acetylcholine receptor • Acetylcholinesterase

KEY POINTS

- Congenital myathenic syndromes refer to a growing list of rare genetic syndromes with abnormal neuromuscular transmission.
- Mutations within the acetylcholine receptor may result in early closure of the channel, prolonged closure of the channel, or a relative deficiency of the channel.
- Mutation in postsynaptic proteins may affect acetylcholine receptor distribution along the postsynaptic membrane.
- Mutations in the acetylcholinesterase proteins can result in prolonged acetylcholine receptor activation.
- Appropriate treatment depends on the specific genetic syndrome of the individual patient.

INTRODUCTION

The congenital myasthenic syndromes (CMS) constitute a growing list of rare genetic conditions that are characterized by abnormal neuromuscular transmission (reviewed in Ref.[1]). The functionally abnormal protein affects the physiology of neurotransmission that often results in fluctuating or fatiguable weakness. The most common forms of CMS are due to mutations in the genes coding for the different subunits of acetylcholine receptor (AChR); these were the first form of CMS to be described in the literature. Subsequently, other forms of CMS have been identified, including mutations coding for (1) proteins in postsynaptic terminal including AChR subunits and other proteins responsible for AChR development and maintenance (including AChR clustering)

Disclosure Statement: P.B. Shieh has served as a consultant for Biogen and Sarepta and a speaker for Biogen and Alexion. He has also received research funding from Sarepta, Ionis, Biogen, PTC, Avexis, Ultragenyx, Pfizer, Catalyst, Roche, BMS, Acceleron, Santhera, Sanofi, Summit, Audentes, Italfarmaco, FibroGen, Reata, and Catabasis. S.J. Oh has no conflict of interest to report.

[a] Department of Neurology, University of California, Los Angeles, 300 Medical Plaza, Suite B-200, Los Angeles, CA 90095, USA; [b] Department of Neurology, University of Alabama at Birmingham, 619 19th Street South, Birmingham, AL 35233, USA
* Corresponding author.
E-mail address: pshieh@mednet.ucla.edu

Neurol Clin 36 (2018) 367–378
https://doi.org/10.1016/j.ncl.2018.01.007
0733-8619/18/© 2018 Elsevier Inc. All rights reserved.

neurologic.theclinics.com

at the endplate, (2) proteins within the synaptic cleft, and (3) presynaptic terminal proteins. **Fig. 1** illustrates this classification scheme. Several of these conditions affect the expression or function of the AChR, and thus the symptoms may be similar to myasthenia gravis. More recently, newer DNA sequencing techniques allow for massively parallel sequencing, resulting in the discovery of newer genetic entities that affect neuromuscular transmission. Some of these conditions affect multiple organ systems and may also affect proteins that span different sites within the neuromuscular junction.

The physiologic basis for most of these syndromes is the reduced response of the postsynaptic terminal to the signal that is entering the presynaptic terminal. The fidelity of this system is typically directly related to the severity of the symptoms the patients experience. In this review, the authors discuss some of the most common forms of CMS.

CLINICAL FEATURES

In most forms of CMS, the symptoms start at birth by definition, but some patients are evaluated later in childhood or early adult life because the symptoms are mild or not recognized. A positive family history is consistent with the diagnosis of CMS, but a negative family history does not exclude autosomal recessive CMS or even dominant inheritance. Most cases of CMS are inherited by an autosomal recessive pattern except one: the classic slow channel syndrome. On examination, the most important clue is increasing weakness on sustained exertion (myasthenic weakness) involving ocular, bulbar, and limb muscles. There are some findings suggestive of specific forms of CMS: scoliosis and delayed pupillary light reflex in acetylcholinesterase collagen tail (ColQ) syndrome, selective severe weakness of cervical muscles and of wrist and

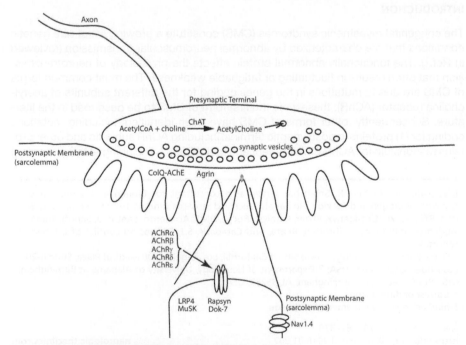

Fig. 1. CMS classified by location of the defective protein.

finger extensor muscles in endplate ColQ syndrome and slow channel syndrome, and lack of ocular muscle involvement in ColQ syndrome, slow channel syndrome, or choline acetyl transferase (ChAT) syndrome.

DIAGNOSIS AND TESTING

Diagnosis of CMS can be made on the basis of the classic tetrad: myasthenic symptoms since birth, exertion-induced weakness on examination, negative AChR and Muscle Specific Kinase (MuSK antibodies), and decremental response at low-rate stimulation in the repetitive nerve stimulation (RNS) test.[2] For the diagnosis of a specific type of CMS, a clinician considers genetic testing for CMS. Genetic testing including expanded panels or those that use next-generation sequencing, however, may not yield a specific diagnosis because patients may have a CMS diagnosis with mutations in genes that have not yet been identified. With increased awareness and improved diagnostic methods, the diagnostic yield of patients with CMS has improved in recent years.

Electrodiagnostic Testing

Diagnosis of CMS is supported by a decremental response at low-rate stimulation in the RNS test or by abnormal jitter and blocking on Single Fiber electromyography (SFEMG).[3] The decremental response at low-rate stimulation in at least one muscle is the most common finding in CMS (**Fig. 2**). When the RNS is normal, usually the SFEMG is abnormal showing abnormal jitters and blocking. The decremental response may be absent in ChAT between attacks. In these cases a decremental response can be elicited by prolonged 10-Hz stimulation or by exercise for several minutes before 2-Hz stimulation. Repetitive discharges, a second peak on the compound motor action potential (CMAP) with a single stimulus, are typically observed in 2 syndromes: ColQ and slow channel syndrome due to "prolonged activation of postsynaptic membrane" (too much ACh) (**Fig. 3**).[4,5]

Genetic Testing

Traditionally, genetic testing was performed using Sanger sequencing, which is directed at single genes and performed with relatively high accuracy. This method is still used when only one genetic entity is suspected (eg, familial testing, confirmatory testing). More recently, massively parallel testing (ie, next-generation sequencing) has been used as a cost-effective method to screen multiple genes when this approach is clinically appropriate. Although there are limitations to these newer techniques, they have significantly improved the ability to diagnose genetic diseases, particularly in patients with rare conditions that are often not suspected, including many of the CMS diagnoses.

A CMS-specific next-generation-sequencing panel can be used by clinicians who are suspecting CMS clinically; not infrequently, however, CMS is identified on whole-exome sequencing because CMS was not suspected. Sometimes, testing will identify variants of unclear significance. Clinical and electrodiagnostic testing may be necessary to confirm the diagnosis of CMS in these cases. Fortunately, specific genes are identified in many CMS, and such a test is now commercially available.

SPECIFIC GENETIC SYNDROMES
Presynaptic

Choline acetyl transferase
Mutations within the gene coding for the ChAT protein result in impaired synthesis of acetylcholine. ChAT is an enzyme in the presynaptic terminal that catalyzes the synthesis of acetylcholine. The relative deficiency of this enzyme leads to relative

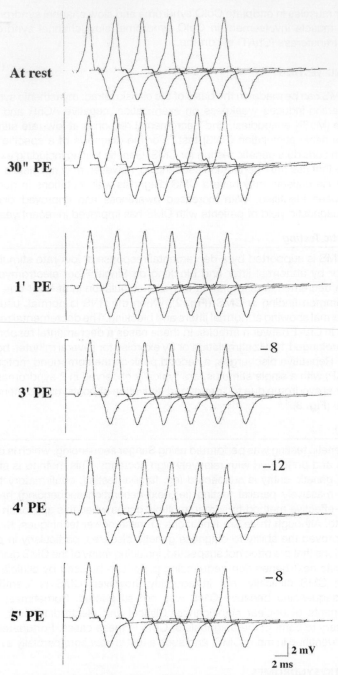

Fig. 2. Postexercise exhaustion (−8 to −12% decrement) in 3-Hz RNS response in the ADM muscle following Lambert's method in a case of postsynaptic anticholinesterase responsive CMS.

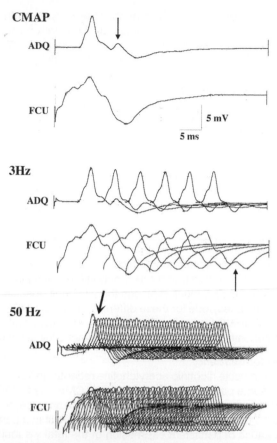

Fig. 3. RNS response in the ADQ (ADM) muscle and flexor carpi ulnaris (FCU) muscles in a case of slow channel syndrome. Repetitive discharge (*thin arrow*) in the CMAP. Decremental response at low-rate stimulation (3 Hz). Dip phenomenon (*thick arrow*) at high-rate stimulation (50 Hz).

depletion of acetylcholine-containing vesicles, which is particularly apparent after prolonged subtetanic stimulation.[6]

The clinical spectrum of patients with ChAT deficiency varies significantly. Some patients are severely affected, presenting at birth with episodic severe apnea and bulbar weakness and ventilator dependence.[7,8] Others may present with mild fixed weakness with occasional apneic episodes, which may be severe.[9] There are also a group of milder patients who present with minimal or no respiratory symptoms and proximal weakness.[8] These patients do improve with acetylcholinesterase inhibitors, and weakness and apnea can be worsened or triggered by cold temperatures, which has not been observed in other myasthenic syndromes.[8] Low-frequency (2 Hz) RNS may be normal, but repeat testing after stimulating at 10 Hz for 5 to 10 minutes will often show a decremental response.

Synaptic

Acetylcholinesterase
The acetylcholinesterase complex comprises catalytic units (AchE) that bind to collagenic tails (ColQ). The catalytic subunits are tetramers of AChE, and the collagenic tail

peptide forms a triple helix that serves to anchor the enzyme to the synaptic cleft. Thus, up to 3 catalytic units bind to a collagenic tail triple helix.[5] The *COLQ* gene encodes the collagenic tail that mediates binding to the synaptic cleft. Thus, mutations in *COLQ* result in mislocalization of AChR enzymatic activity, which results in a deficiency of acetylcholinesterase within the synaptic cleft.

Patients with severe ColQ deficiency may present during infancy with severe axial weakness. Patients with milder ColQ deficiency may present in childhood, and extraocular muscles may be spared. Severely affected patients may demonstrate a slowed pupillary response to light.[5] Because of prolonged activation of the postsynaptic membrane, a second peak on the compound muscle action potential may be observed with a single stimulus[4,5] (see **Fig. 3**). This second peak (repetitive CMAP) should attenuate rapidly with 2- to 3-Hz RNS. Cholinesterase inhibitors (eg, pyridostigmine) are contraindicated in patients with ColQ deficiency. Patients, however, may benefit from adrenergic agonists such as ephedrine or albuterol.[10–12]

Postsynaptic

Acetylcholine receptor

The muscle nicotinic AChR is a pentamer, which, in the fetal form, consists of 2 α subunits, one β subunit, one δ subunit, and one γ subunit, resulting in a stoichiometry of $\alpha_2\beta\delta\gamma$. In the adult form, the ε subunit replaces the γ subunit, resulting in a stoichiometry of $\alpha_2\beta\delta\varepsilon$. Different genes code for these different subunits: *CHRNA1* for α, *CHRNB* for β, *CHRND* for δ, *CHRNG* for γ, and *CHRNE* for ε. Mutations within the genes that code the different subunits may result in several distinct clinical syndromes.[13]

Acetylcholine receptor deficiency

Relative reduction in muscle nicotinic acetylcholine receptor (nAChR-muscle) expression is observed in some patients and is classified as CMS due to "AChR deficiency." Most commonly, this form of CMS is autosomal recessive and due to a null mutation in the CHRNE gene.[14,15] These mutations, however, only result in a partial deficiency of nAChR-muscle because of persistent expression of the fetal γ subunit, which serves to rescue/replace the deficient ε subunit. Null mutations in the other subunits would result in complete deficiency of the nAChR-muscle because those subunits do not have fetal isoforms that would partially rescue their function. These mutations have not been observed and are likely embryonically lethal. A 2- to 3-Hz RNS of a patient with symptomatic AChR deficiency would likely result in a decremental response pattern. Patients may benefit from treatments that increase AChR activation, including AChE inhibitors (eg, pyridostigmine) and/or 3,4-Diaminopyridine (3,4-DAP).

Slow channel syndrome

Mutations resulting in prolonged activation of the AChR are classified as slow channel syndrome. This form of CMS is the result of autosomal dominant gain-of-function mutations affecting the pore and ligand binding regions.[16] As with ColQ deficiency, prolonged activation of the postsynaptic membrane in slow channel syndrome often results in a repetitive (second) compound muscle action potential with a single stimulus on electrodiagnostic testing (see **Fig. 3**). RNS at 2 to 3 Hz of a patient with symptomatic slow channel will likely demonstrate a decremental response. A repetitive CMAP can be observed in patients with slow channel syndrome and this second peak should attenuate rapidly with 2- to 3-Hz RNS (see **Fig. 3**). Cholinesterase inhibitors (eg, pyridostigmine) and other agents designed to increase AChR activation (eg, 3,4-DAP) are contraindicated in patients with slow channel syndrome. Patients, however, may benefit from quinidine[17] or fluoxetine,[18–20] which appear to block open AChR channels and minimize the clinical effects of prolonged AChR opening.

Fast channel syndrome

Mutations that result in shortened time of opening of the AChR pore are classified as "fast channel" mutations. The fast channel syndrome is autosomal recessive and may be the result of a compound heterozygous combination of a fast channel mutation paired with a null mutation. Multiple mutations in the α, δ, and ε subunits have been described and generally fall into 4 categories: (1) mutations that change the AChR affinity for acetylcholine,[21] (2) mutations that interfere with activation,[22] (3) mutations that change gating efficiency,[23] and (4) mutations within ε that reduce the stability of the activated receptor.[24] Two- to 3-Hz RNS of a patient with symptomatic fast channel syndrome would likely result in a decremental response pattern, and patients may benefit from treatments that increase AChR activation (eg, pyridostigmine and/or 3,4-DAP).

Dok-7 (DOK7)

Defects in the Dok-7 protein were suspected to cause CMS based on Dok-7's interaction with MuSK. Patients that were suspected of CMS were subsequently found to have mutation in the *DOK7* gene,[25] and patients across a clinical spectrum have subsequently been described.[26–28]

Patients with *DOK7*-associated CMS are generally found to have weakness affecting the limb-girdle distribution more prominently than in the ocular-bulbar distribution. Two- to 3-Hz RNS would result in a decremental response pattern. Patients, however, do not respond to agents to increase AChR activation (eg, pyridostigmine and/or 3,4-DAP), but appear to respond to adrenergic agonists such as ephedrine or albuterol.[12,29,30]

Rapsyn (RAPSN)

Mutations in *RAPSN* were described in patients with CMS characterized by a deficiency of AChR channels.[31] A functional deficiency of AChR would fit with the role of the Rapsyn protein in the clustering of AChR channels in the postsynaptic membrane.[32] More recently, *RAPSN* mutations have been described across a phenotypic spectrum, including early-onset congenital forms as well as late-onset patients.[33,34] Clinically significant ophthalmoplegia is not associated with *RAPSN* CMS. Late-onset patients may be misdiagnosed with seronegative myasthenia gravis,[33] and the late-onset limb-girdle pattern may even be misdiagnosed with muscular dystrophy. Many patients with CMS of European descent may carry the N88K founder mutation,[35] and another specific founder mutation, c.−38A>G, which is within the E-box region, has been described in the Middle Eastern Jewish population with mild bulbar and facial weakness.[36] Otherwise, there are no specific genotype-phenotype correlations. Two- to 3-Hz RNS often results in a decremental response pattern. Patients with Rapsyn typically report a response to a combination of pyridostigmine and 3,4-DAP[37]; ephedrine or albuterol may provide additional benefit.[37]

Na_v1.4 (SCN4A)

CMS may also be associated with mutations in *SCN4A*, which encodes $Na_v1.4$, the common voltage gated sodium channel in muscle. These mutations have been described in 2 patients that presented with fluctuating/episodic weakness involving limbs, axial musculature, and respiratory muscles.[38,39] There was some response to pyridostigmine[38,39] and possibly acetazolamide.[38]

SCN4A is more commonly associated with autosomal dominant periodic paralysis and potassium-aggravated myotonia. These syndromes are due to either a gain of function mutation or a dominant negative mutation in this sodium channel (reviewed in Ref.[40]). In contrast, the CMS mutations are presumed to result from loss of function of this protein and would thus predict an autosomal recessive condition with attenuated activation of the postsynaptic membrane.[39,40] Thus, physiologically, these synapses are exhibiting diminished activation that may be characterized as a myasthenic syndrome.

Congenital myasthenic syndromes and other postsynaptic proteins

Antibodies against MuSK (*MUSK*) and Lrp4 (*LRP4*) have been associated with rare forms of myasthenia gravis. Thus, the role of these proteins in neuromuscular transmission can be easily inferred. Agrin (*AGRN*) is a protein that is secreted by the presynaptic terminal during development and binds to Lrp4 on the postsynaptic membrane. Agrin and Lrp4 together then activate MuSK, which in turn modulates a cluster of AChR channels through Dok-7 and Rapsyn (reviewed in Ref.[41]; for more detailed discussion, the reader is referred to Hiroshi Nishimune and Kazuhiro Shigemoto's article, "Practical Anatomy of the Neuromuscular Junction in Health and Disease," and Robert L. Ruff and Robert P. Lisak's article, "Nature and Action of Antibodies in Myasthenia Gravis," in this issue). Although agrin is expressed by the presynaptic terminal, the effect of *AGRN* mutations would predominantly affect the postsynaptic terminal. Thus, it can also be grouped with the postsynaptic proteins.

Mutations in *AGRN*, *MUSK*, and *LRP4* have all been described to cause CMS, although only in a handful of patients for *AGRN*[42,43] and *MUSK*[44,45] and only in one patient for *LRP4*.[46] Albuterol may be helpful in patients with *MUSK* mutation,[47] but it is unclear what treatments would benefit patients with mutations in *AGRN* or *LRP4*.

Other Genes That Result in Congenital Myasthenic Syndromes

A growing list of CMS genes have been reported, including conditions that overlap with myopathies. For example, some of the centronuclear myopathies syndromes have clinical symptoms and electrophysiological findings that, at some level, are consistent with a defect of neuromuscular transmission. These centronuclear myopathies include the syndromes associated with mutations in *BIN1*,[48] *MTM1*,[49] and *DNM2*,[50] and some of these patients have exhibited a mild response to pyridostigmine. Thus, these patients appear to have a CMS-myopathy overlap. In addition, laminin β-2 (*LAMB2*)[51] and Plectin (*PLEC*)[52,53] have been reported to have electrophysiological findings consistent with impaired neuromuscular transmission. These mutations may have multisystem involvement, including the ocular and renal abnormalities reported in the *LAMB2* patient and epidermolysis bullosa simplex with muscular dystrophy in *PLEC* patients.[54]

Patients with a certain congenital defect of glycosylation have also been classified as having a form of CMS. In particular, patients with mutation in *GFPT1*[55] have been described to have limb-girdle distribution of weakness that is mildly responsive to pyridostigmine. The pathophysiology appears to be that of altered glycosylation of synaptic proteins, resulting in impaired neuromuscular transmission. Other genes associated with congenital defects of glycosylation have also been proposed to affect neuromuscular transmission, including mutations in *DPAGT1* that may also be associated with intellectual disability.[56]

TREATMENT

As described through this review, various different symptomatic treatments have been tried for each of the different CMS syndromes (**Table 1**). Clinical trials for these rare conditions are unlikely to recruit many patients, and thus, literature based on empiric treatment of individual cases or case series continue to the main source of guidance for the treatment of CMS. For most of the CMS syndromes that can be characterized physiologically as having "underactive" synapses, a trial of an AChE inhibitor and/or 3,4-DAP may be appropriate. The exception is Dok-7; these patients do not respond

Table 1
Treatment of some of the more common congenital myasthenic syndromes

Location	Syndrome	Inheritance	Treatment	Comments
Presynaptic	ChAT	Recessive	AChE inhibitor	Consider ventilator & apnea monitor
Synaptic	ColQ	Recessive	β-Agonist	AChE inhibitors contraindicated
Postsynaptic	AChR deficiency	Recessive	AChE inhibitor, 3,4-DAP	Consider β-agonist
	Slow channel	Dominant	Fluoxetine, quinidine	AChE inhibitors contraindicated
	Fast channel	Recessive	AChE inhibitor, 3,4-DAP	
	Dok-7	Recessive	β-Agonist	AChE inhibitors contraindicated
	Rapsyn	Recessive	AChE inhibitor, 3,4-DAP	Consider β-agonist
	GFPT1	Recessive	AChE inhibitor, 3,4-DAP	

to AChE inhibitors,[44] which may be reminiscent of patients with anti-MuSK myasthenia gravis who do not respond to AChE inibitors.[57] Some of the CMS syndromes can be described physiologically as having "overactive" synapses (eg, ColQ deficiency and slow channel syndrome). In these cases, AChE inhibitors are contraindicated. Patients with slow channel syndrome may benefit from treatment of long-acting agents that block the AChR channel, such as quinidine or fluoxetine. Finally, albuterol or one of the β-agonists have been empirically found to benefit patients with Dok-7 and ColQ deficiency and may be considered in some of the other syndromes as well.

SUMMARY

The CMS are a group of conditions that result from impaired neuromuscular transmission. Genes associated with CMS are expressed in the synapse, on either the presynaptic membrane, synaptic cleft, or postsynaptic membrane. The clinical diagnosis is often made based on early onset of fluctuating and/or fatiguable weakness that can be confirmed by electrodiagnostic testing. Many patients, however, will still remain undiagnosed even when in the care of experienced clinicians. Confirmatory genetic testing can be challenging, especially with conditions where the genetic correlation is less established. The CMS group continues to be an extremely rare condition, but as more cases are recognized and reported, awareness among clinicians will improve, laboratory testing will become more available, and treatments will become better characterized.

REFERENCES

1. Engel AG, Shen XM, Selcen D, et al. Congenital myasthenic syndromes: pathogenesis, diagnosis, and treatment. Lancet Neurol 2015;14:420–34.
2. Engel AG. Congenital myasthenic syndrome. Neurol Clin 1994;12(2):401–37.
3. Kimura J. Electrodiagnosis in disease of nerve and muscle: principles and practice. 3rd edition. Oxford University; 1989.
4. Engel AG, Lambert EH, Gomez MR. A new myasthenic syndrome with end-plate acetylcholinesterase deficiency, small nerve terminals, and reduced acetylcholine release. Ann Neurol 1977;1:315–30.
5. Hutchinson DO, Walls TJ, Nakano S, et al. Congenital endplate acetylcholinesterase deficiency. Brain 1993;116:633–53.

6. Ohno K, Tsujino A, Shen XM, et al. Choline acetyltransferase mutations cause myasthenic syndrome associated with episodic apnea in humans. Proc Natl Acad Sci U S A 2001;98:2017–22.
7. Byring RF, Pihko H, Shen XM, et al. Congenital myasthenic syndrome associated with episodic apnea and sudden infant death. Neuromuscul Disord 2002;12: 548–53.
8. Maselli RA, Chen D, Mo D, et al. Choline acetyltransferase mutations in myasthenic syndrome due to deficient acetylcholine resynthesis. Muscle Nerve 2003;27:180–7.
9. Schara U, Christen HJ, Durmus H, et al. Long-term follow-up in patients with congenital myasthenic syndrome due to CHAT mutations. Eur J Paediatr Neurol 2010;14:326–33.
10. Bestue-Cardiel M, de-Cabazon-Alvarez AS, Capablo-Liesa JL, et al. Congenital endplate acetylcholinesterase deficiency responsive to ephedrine. Neurology 2005;65:144–6.
11. Mihaylova V, Muller JS, Vilchez JJ, et al. Clinical and molecular genetic findings in COLQ-mutant congenital myasthenic syndromes. Brain 2008;131:747–59.
12. Liewluck T, Selcen D, Engel AG. Beneficial effects of albuterol in congenital end-plate acetylcholinesterase deficiency and DOK-7 myasthenia. Muscle Nerve 2011;44:789–94.
13. Unwin N. Structure and action of the nicotinic acetylcholine receptor explored by electron microscopy. FEBS Lett 2003;555:91–5.
14. Engel AG, Ohno K, Bouzat C, et al. End-plate acetylcholine receptor deficiency due to nonsense mutations in the ε subunit. Ann Neurol 1996;40:810–7.
15. Ohno K, Quiram P, Milone M, et al. Congenital myasthenic syndromes due to heteroallelic nonsense/missense mutations in the acetylcholine receptor ε subunit gene: identification and functional characterization of six new mutations. Hum Mol Genet 1997;6:753–66.
16. Ohno K, Hutchinson DO, Milone M, et al. Congenital myasthenic syndrome caused by prolonged acetylcholine receptor channel openings due to a mutation in the M2 domain of the ε subunit. Proc Natl Acad Sci USA 1995;92:758–62.
17. Harper CM, Engel AG. Quinidine sulfate therapy for the slow-channel congenital myasthenic syndrome. Ann Neurol 1998;43:480–4.
18. Harper CM, Fukudome T, Engel AG. Treatment of slow channel congenital myasthenic syndrome with fluoxetine. Neurology 2003;60:170–3.
19. Colomer J, Muller JS, Vernet A, et al. Long-term improvement of slow-channel myasthenic syndrome with fluoxetine. Neuromuscul Disord 2006;16:329–33.
20. Chaouch A, Muller JS, Guergueltcheva V, et al. A retrospective clinical study of the slow-channel congenital myasthenic syndrome. J Neurol 2012;259:474–81.
21. Shen XM, Brengman J, Edvardson S, et al. Highly fatal fast-channel congenital syndrome caused by AChR ε subunit mutation at the agonist binding site. Neurology 2012;79:449–54.
22. Shen XM, Ohno K, Tsujino A, et al. Mutation causing severe myasthenia reveals functional asymmetry of AChR signature Cys-loops in agonist binding and gating. J Clin Invest 2003;111:497–505.
23. Wang HL, Milone M, Ohno K, et al. Acetylcholine receptor M3 domain: stereochemical and volume contributions to channel gating. Nat Neurosci 1999;2: 226–33.
24. Wang HL, Ohno K, Milone M, et al. Fundamental gating mechanism of nicotinic receptor channel revealed by mutation causing a congenital myasthenic syndrome. J Gen Physiol 2000;116:449–60.

25. Beeson D, Higuchi O, Palace J, et al. Dok-7 mutations underlie a neuromuscular junction synaptopathy. Science 2006;313:1975–8.
26. Muller JS, Herczegfalvi A, Vilchez JJ, et al. Phenotypical spectrum of DOK7 mutations in congenital myasthenic syndromes. Brain 2007;130:1497–506.
27. Anderson JA, Ng JJ, Bowe C, et al. Variable phenotypes associated with mutations in *DOK7*. Muscle Nerve 2008;37:448–56.
28. Ammar AB, Petit F, Alexandri K, et al. Phenotype-genotype analysis in 15 patients presenting a congenital myasthenic syndrome due to mutations in *DOK7*. J Neurol 2010;257:754–66.
29. Selcen D, Milone M, Shen XM, et al. Dok-7 myasthenia: phenotypic and molecular genetic studies in 16 patients. Ann Neurol 2008;64:71–87.
30. Schara U, Barisic N, Deschauer M, et al. Ephedrine therapy in eight patients with congenital myasthenic syndrome due to *DOK7* mutations. Neuromuscul Disord 2010;19:828–32.
31. Ohno K, Engel AG, Shen XM, et al. Rapsyn mutations in humans cause endplate acetylcholine receptor deficiency and myasthenic syndrome. Am J Hum Genet 2002;70:875–85.
32. Ramarao MK, Cohen JB. Mechanism of nicotinic acetylcholine receptor cluster formation by rapsyn. Proc Natl Acad Sci USA 1998;95:4007–12.
33. Burke G, Cossins J, Maxwell S, et al. Rapsyn mutations in hereditary myasthenia. Distinct early- and late-onset phenotypes. Neurology 2003;61:826–8.
34. Milone M, Shen XM, Selcen D, et al. Myasthenic syndrome due to defects in rapsyn: clinical and molecular findings in 39 patients. Neurology 2009;73:228–35.
35. Müller JS, Mildner G, Müller-Felber W, et al. Rapsyn N88K is a frequent cause of CMS in European patients. Neurology 2003;60:1805–11.
36. Ohno K, Sadoh M, Blatt I, et al. E-box mutations in RAPSN promoter region in eight cases with congenital myasthenic syndrome. Hum Mol Genet 2003;12: 739–48.
37. Banwell BL, Ohno K, Sieb JP, et al. Novel truncating *RAPSN* mutation causing congenital myasthenic syndrome responsive to 3,4-diaminopyridine. Neuromuscul Disord 2004;14:202–7.
38. Tsujino A, Maertens C, Ohno K, et al. Myasthenic syndrome caused by mutation of the *SCN4A* sodium channel. Proc Natl Acad Sci USA 2003;100:7377–82.
39. Habbout K, Poulin H, Rivier F, et al. A recessive Na$_v$1.4 mutation underlies congenital myasthenic syndrome with periodic paralysis. Neurology 2016;86: 161–9.
40. Nicole S, Fontaine B. Skeletal muscle sodium channelopathies. Curr Opin Neurol 2015;8:508–14.
41. Burden SJ, Yumoto N, Zhang W. The role of MuSK in synapse formation and neuromuscular disease. Cold Spring Harb Perspect Biol 2013;5:a009167.
42. Huze C, Bauche S, Richard P, et al. Identification of an agrin mutation that causes congenital myasthenia and affects synapse function. Am J Hum Genet 2009;85: 155–67.
43. Maselli RA, Fernandez JM, Arredondo J, et al. LG2 agrin mutation causing severe congenital myasthenic syndrome mimics functional characteristics of non-neural agrin (z-) agrin. Hum Genet 2012;131:1123–35.
44. Chevessier F, Faraut B, Ravel-Chapuis A, et al. MUSK, a new target for mutations causing congenital myasthenic syndrome. Hum Mol Genet 2004;13:3229–40.
45. Mihaylova V, Salih MA, Mukhtar MM, et al. Refinement of the clinical phenotype in MUSK-related congenital myasthenic syndromes. Neurology 2009;73:1926–8.

46. Ohkawara B, Cabrera-Serrano M, Nakat T, et al. LRP4 third β-propeller domain mutations cause novel congenital myasthenic syndrome by compromising agrin-mediated MuSK signalling in a position-specific manner. Hum Mol Genet 2014;23:1856–68.

47. Gallenmuller C, Muller-Felber W, Dusl M, et al. Salbutamol-responsive limb-girdle congenital myasthenic syndrome due to a novel missense mutation and hetero-allelic deletion in MUSK. Neuromuscul Disord 2014;24:31–5.

48. Claeys KG, Maisonobe T, Bohm J, et al. Phenotype of a patient with recessive centronuclear myopathy and a novel BIN1 mutation. Neurology 2010;74:519–21.

49. Robb SA, Sewry CA, Dowling JJ, et al. Impaired neuromuscular transmission and response to aceylcholinesterase inhibitors in centronuclear myopathy. Neuromuscul Disord 2011;21:379–86.

50. Gibbs EM, Clarke NF, Rose K, et al. Neuromuscular junction abnormalities in DNM2-related centronuclear myopathy. J Mol Med (Berl) 2013;91:727–37.

51. Maselli RA, Ng JJ, Andreson JA, et al. Mutations in *LAMB2* causing a severe form of synaptic congenital myasthenic syndrome. J Med Genet 2009;46:203–8.

52. Banwell BL, Russel J, Fukudome T, et al. Myopathy, myasthenic syndrome, and epidermolysis bullosa simplex due to plectin deficiency. J Neuropathol Exp Neurol 1999;58:832–46.

53. Selcen D, Juel VC, Hobson-Webb LD, et al. Myasthenic syndrome caused by plectinopathy. Neurology 2011;76:327–36.

54. McMillan JR, Akiyama M, Rouan F, et al. Plectin defects in epidermolysis bullosa simplex with muscular dystrophy. Muscle Nerve 2007;35:24–35.

55. Senderek J, Muller JS, Dusl M, et al. Hexosamine biosynthetic pathway mutations cause neuromuscular transmission defect. Am J Hum Genet 2011;88:162–72.

56. Selcen D, Shen XM, Li Y, et al. DPAGT1 myasthenia and myopathy. Genetic, phenotypic, and expression studies. Neurology 2014;82:1822–30.

57. Hatanaka Y, Hemmi S, Morgan MG, et al. Nonresponsiveness to anticholinesterase agents in pateints with MuSK-antibody positive MG. Neurology 2005;65:1508–9.

Lambert-Eaton Myasthenic Syndrome

Vita G. Kesner, MD, PhD[a],*, Shin J. Oh, MD[b], Mazen M. Dimachkie, MD[c],
Richard J. Barohn, MD[c]

KEYWORDS

- Lambert-Eaton myasthenic syndrome • Neuromuscular transmission disorder
- Paraneoplastic syndrome • P/Q-type voltage-gated calcium channels
- 3,4-Diaminopyridine

KEY POINTS

- LEMS is a paraneoplastic or primary autoimmune neuromuscular junction disorder. The antigenic target is the P/Q-type voltage-gated calcium channel (VGCC), which plays a role in decreasing the release of acetylcholine.
- The clinical triad typically consists of proximal muscle weakness, autonomic features, and areflexia.
- Characteristic electrophysiologic triads are the low compound muscle action potentials (CMAP), decremental response at the low-rate stimulation, and incremental response with 10 seconds maximal voluntary contraction or high-rate stimulation.
- Paraneoplastic form of LEMS occurs almost always with an underlying small cell lung cancer (SCLC). Cancer screening should continue every 3 to 6 months for at least 2 years from symptom onset.
- Effective symptomatic treatment of LEMS is with 3,4-diaminopyridine.

Disclosures: Dr. M.M. Dimachkie is on the speaker's bureau or is a consultant for Alnylam, Baxalta, Catalyst, CSLBehring, Mallinckrodt, Novartis, NuFactor, and Terumo. He has also received grants from Alexion, Biomarin, Catalyst, CSL Behring, FDA/OPD, GSK, Grifols, MDA, NIH, Novartis, Orphazyme, Sanofi, and TMA. Dr R.J. Barohn is a consultant for NuFactor and is on the advisory board for Novartis. He has received an honorarium from Option Care and PlatformQ Health Education. He has received research grants from NIH, FDA/OOPD, NINDS, Novartis, Sanofi/Genzyme, Biomarin, IONIS, Teva, Cytokinetics, Eli Lilly, PCORI, ALSA, and PTC. This work was supported by a CTSA grant from NCATS awarded to the University of Kansas for Frontiers: University of Kansas Clinical and Translational Science Institute (# UL1TR002366) The contents are solely the responsibility of the authors and do not necessarily represent the official views of the NIH or NCATS.
a Neurology Department, 12 Executive Park Drive NE, Atlanta, GA 30329, USA; b University of Alabama at Birmingham, Department of Neurology, SC 350, 1720 2nd Ave South, Birmingham, AL 35294, USA; c Department of Neurology, University of Kansas Medical Center, 3901 Rainbow Boulevard, Mail Stop 2012, Kansas City, KS 66160, USA
* Corresponding author.
E-mail address: vkesner@emory.edu

INTRODUCTION

The Lambert-Eaton myasthenic syndrome (LEMS) is a paraneoplastic or primary auto-immune neuromuscular junction disorder characterized by proximal weakness and autonomic dysfunction. The characteristic weakness is thought to be caused by anti-bodies generated against the P/Q-type voltage-gated calcium channels (VGCC) present on presynaptic nerve terminals and by diminished release of acetylcholine (ACh). More than half of LEMS cases are associated with small cell lung carcinoma (SCLC), which expresses functional VGCC. Diagnosis is confirmed by serologic testing and electrophysiologic studies.

HISTORICAL NOTE

In 1953, Anderson and colleagues[1] described a 47-year-old man with fatigable proximal weakness, dysphasia, and diminished Deep Tendon Reflex (DTRs) who improved after an oat cell (small cell) lung cancer was surgically removed. At a meeting of the American Physiologic Society in 1956, Lambert and coworkers[2] presented a report on six patients with defective neuromuscular transmission associated with malignant neoplasms. They identified some of the clinical and electrophysiologic features that were different from what were expected in typical myasthenia gravis (MG). Subsequently, in 1957, Eaton and Lambert[3] reported the distinctive electrophysiologic abnormalities seen with repetitive nerve stimulation (RNS) and identified a syndrome that has become known as LEMS. The diagnosis is still based on these electrophysiologic criteria. Soon after the original report, two publications[4,5] from the same department highlighted the range of clinical and electrophysiologic features of this syndrome in 30 patients, including patients without lung cancer. The calcium channels as a target of the pathogenic antibodies in LEMS were first suggested by Fukunaga and colleagues[6] in 1983. The discovery of pathogenic autoantibodies to VGCC has facilitated diagnosis and improved the understanding of the pathophysiologic mechanisms leading to LEMS (1983–1995). Subsequent studies showed antibodies against P/Q-type calcium channel as the most prominent in these patients.[7] Over the past decade, knowledge of epidemiologic and clinical features of LEMS has expanded.

EPIDEMIOLOGY

LEMS is a rare disorder with annual incidence of only one-tenth to one-fourteenth of that of MG with a prevalence that is 46 times less than that of MG.[8] Sanders[9] estimated the prevalence of LEMS in the United States to be 1 in 100,000 on the basis of prevalence of small cell lung cancer. In the paraneoplastic form of the disease (SCLC-LEMS) the median age at onset is 60 years and 65% to 75% of patients are men.[10] The age and sex distribution in nontumor LEMS (NT-LEMS) is similar to that reported for MG. NT-LEMS is seen at all ages, with a peak age of onset of around 35 years and a second, larger peak at age 60 years. Most patients with NT-LEMS are female.[10,11] The genetic association with HLA-B8-DR3 haplotype is linked to autoimmunity and is present in around 65% of patients with young onset of NT-LEMS.[12]

TUMOR ASSOCIATION AND IMMUNOPATHOPHYSIOLOGY

Tumor association is reported in about 60% of patients with LEMS.[11] Most patients have SCLC, a smoking-related lung carcinoma with neuroendocrine characteristics, but other malignancies have been described (non–small cell and mixed lung carcinomas, prostate carcinoma, thymoma, and lymphoproliferative disorders).[11,13,14] The diagnosis of LEMS usually precedes the diagnosis of cancer by many months and even up to 2 years. In a large study of 227 patients, the diagnosis of cancer ranged from 5 years before to 6 years after onset of LEMS.[11] Weight loss, being male, and a history of smoking are considered to be risk factors. Patients with SCLC associated with LEMS live longer than patients with similar lung cancer stage without a paraneoplastic disorder. An effective immune response directed against cancer is thought to be responsible for this phenomenon.[13]

The initial humoral autoimmune response in patients with LEMS is assumed to be generated against the VGCC subunit antigens on the lung carcinoma.[7,15] SCLC expresses VGCC of the N, L, or P type.[16] VGCC of the P/Q (VGCC-P/Q) and possibly N (VGCC-N) types are targets of IgG-mediated nerve terminal autoimmunity in LEMS.[17] P/Q-type VGCCs are involved in ACh release from adult mammalian motor nerve terminals and N-type is responsible for transmitter release from peripheral autonomic nerve terminals.[18,19]

The patient's IgG injected into mice transmits the microelectrophysiologic and ultrastructural changes associated with the disease. Structural alteration of calcium-channel–enriched presynaptic membranes and disruption by LEMS-patient serum of depolarization-dependent Ca influx in cultured small cell carcinoma cells and murine motor nerve terminals were noted on electron microscopy.[6,20] VGCC antibodies block the ability of calcium to flow into the nerve terminal when depolarization occurs, which causes a disruption in the release of ACh. This, in turn, leads to a reduced number of contracting muscles fibers and subsequent weakness.

CLINICAL FEATURES

The clinical triad typically consists of proximal muscle weakness, autonomic features, and areflexia.[14] The onset of symptoms is usually gradual and insidious but occasionally it is subacute. Presenting symptoms are leg weakness (60%), generalized weakness (18%), muscle pain or stiffness (5%), dry mouth (5%), arm weakness (4%), diplopia (4%), and dysarthria (2%).[11] Others have described muscle weakness in 96% of 227 patients with LEMS, mostly of the legs, oculobulbar symptoms in 51%, autonomic symptoms in 49%, respiratory symptoms in 16%, and sensory symptoms in 15%.[11]

Spreading of weakness in patients with NT-LEMS and SCLC-LEMS was described by Titulaer and coworkers.[21] Weakness normally spreads proximally to distally, involving feet and hands, and caudally to cranially, finally reaching the oculobulbar region (Fig. 1). This is in contrast to MG, when weakness typically starts cranially and then descends. The speed of progression is much more pronounced in SCLC-LEMS than in NT-LEMS. At the 3-month mark since the onset of symptoms, patients with SCLC-LEMS had proximal legs and arms weakness (see Fig. 1C) but a large percentage of patients with NT-LEMS had only proximal legs weakness (see Fig. 1A). Occurrence of mild cranial nerve symptoms, including diplopia, ptosis, and dysphagia, ranges from 0% to 80%.[14,22,23] Oculobulbar symptoms and/or signs were present in 78% of patients with LEMS (n = 23) evaluated at the Lahey Clinic.[23] A total of 65% of their patients had ptosis and/or diplopia. In a study of 23 patients with LEMS, bulbar signs and symptoms, including dysarthria, were observed in 10 patients and dysphagia in eight patients. The frequency of ocular and bulbar symptoms in a cohort of 234 patients was reported to be 49% and 52%, respectively, within 12 months of onset (particularly in patients with SCLC-LEMS).[21] A retrospective review of the medical records of all patients diagnosed with LEMS at the Mayo Clinic in Rochester, Minnesota was performed with special attention to ophthalmic symptoms and signs.[24] A total of 176 patients were analyzed with the following findings: ophthalmic symptoms included ptosis in 23%, diplopia in 20.5%, decreased vision in 14%, and dry eye complaints in 7%; ophthalmic

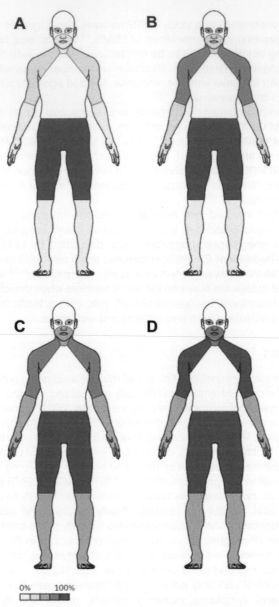

Fig. 1. Spreading of symptoms in patients with NT-LEMS and SCLC-LEMS. Frequency of symptoms at 3 months (*A*) and 12 months (*B*) in patients with NT-LEMS, and frequency of symptoms at 3 months (*C*) and 12 months (*D*) in patients with SCLC-LEMS. The percentages describe the approximate proportion of patients who have that symptom within the given timeframe. (*From* Titulaer MJ, Lang B, Verschuuren JJ. Lambert-Eaton myasthenic syndrome: from clinical characteristics to therapeutic strategies. Lancet Neurol 2011;10(12):1099; Reprinted with permission from Elsevier (The Lancet).)

signs included ptosis in 26%, abnormal ocular motility in 8.5%, strabismus in 8%, pupillary dysfunction in 7%, and findings consistent with dry eyes in 2%. Overall, ocular and bulbar symptoms appear later in the course of the disease of severely affected patients. Although cases of purely ocular symptoms have been reported,[25,26] isolated ocular weakness is extremely rare and ophthalmoplegia on examination is extremely unusual in LEMS. Respiratory failure is infrequent in LEMS and it is often related to the use of paralytic agents or intercurrent pulmonary pathology,[27] but artificial ventilation was reported in up to 11% of cases.[11]

Autonomic dysfunction is reported in 80% to 96% of patients with LEMS.[14,22,28,29] Severe autonomic dysfunction is found on testing even when symptoms are minimal. Both the sympathetic and parasympathetic systems are affected.[30,31]

The most common patient complaint is dry mouth. Other symptoms are erectile dysfunction in men, constipation, orthostatic dysfunction, micturition difficulties, dry eyes, and altered perspiration.[21]

Decreased or absent tendon reflexes are typically seen in patients with LEMS. Postexercise facilitation (a short-term return of tendon reflexes and muscle strength to normal range after muscle contraction) is a characteristic (although not very sensitive) phenomenon, which is present in 40% of patients.[32,33] Tendon reflexes should be tested after a period of rest because postexercise facilitation phenomenon can mask the hypoactive tendon reflexes.

There are reports of patients having both LEMS and MG. Fifty-five possible cases of MG Lambert-Eaton overlap syndrome were identified through PubMed.[34] Thirty-nine cases met the universally accepted diagnostic criteria for MG and LEMS. Analysis of clinical features showed that these patients have common MG and LEMS symptoms: oculobulbar paresis and good response to anticholinesterase for MG and limb weakness and decreased or absent reflexes for LEMS. All patients had the classical LEMS pattern in the RNS test: low compound muscle action potential (CMAP) amplitude and incremental response greater than 60% with brief exercise or at high rate of stimulation. Eight patients had combined positive AChR antibody or muscle-specific kinase antibody and VGCC antibody tests.

DIAGNOSIS

The diagnosis of LEMS is made based on typical clinical features. Confirmation of diagnosis is based on detection of specific VGCC antibodies and characteristic electrodiagnostic findings.

Voltage-Gated Calcium Channels and SOX1 Antibodies

The finding of a high serum titer of antibodies against P/Q-type VGCCs strongly supports the diagnosis of Lambert-Eaton syndrome. P/Q VGCC antibodies are present in 80% to 90% of patients with LEMS.[7,35] P/Q-type VGCCs antibodies have been reported in up to 100% of patients with LEMS who have small cell lung cancer and in up to 90% of patients with LEMS who do not have underlying malignancy. More than 90% of patients belonging to both groups of LEMS (NT-LEMS and SCLC-LEMS) have antibodies against P/Q-type VGCCs.

Antibodies against N-type VGCCs are found more commonly in LEMS associated with primary lung cancer[7] and, accordingly, the detection of N-type antibodies may increase the possibility of finding an underlying malignancy.

Hajela and coworkers[36] reported that multiple components of the presynaptic VGCC complex are prospective targets for antibodies in LEMS. Autoantibodies from patients with LEMS bind directly to multiple VGCC a1 subunits and the b3 subunit.

A total of 10% to 15% of patients with LEMS have no detectable P/Q VGCC antibodies. Possible explanations have been entertained because the antibodies have lower concentration, different epitopes of VGCC, or antibodies to other proteins. Nakao and colleagues[37] studied a cohort (n = 17) of seronegative patients with clinically definite LEMS. The clinical phenotype in this cohort was similar to that in seropositive patients. Incidence of SCLC was only 12%, compared with 60% to 70% in seropositive patients. Electrophysiologic features were similar but less prominent.[38]

VGCC autoimmunity (VGCC-P/Q and VGCC-N types) occurs beyond Lambert–Eaton syndrome and lung cancer. Positive VGCC antibodies were reported in less than 5% of patients with MG and up to 25% of patients with lung cancer without LEMS. Zalewski and colleagues[17] reviewed 236 patients at the Mayo Clinic with VGCC antibodies that were found in evaluation for paraneoplastic neurologic autoimmunity. VGCC autoantibodies were detected in 3.4% of neurologic patients, 1.7% of healthy control subjects, and 4% of neurologically asymptomatic lung cancer control subjects. Twenty-one percent of neurologic patients had more than one neoplasm, historically or detected prospectively (SCLC, breast adenocarcinoma, lymphoma, and suspected tonsillar carcinoma). Autoimmune neurologic diagnosis frequencies, including neuromuscular junction disorder, among patients with medium values (24%; 0.10–0.99 nmol/L) or low values (19%; 0.03–0.10 nmol/L) were fewer than among patients with antibody values exceeding 1.00 nmol/L (71%; $P = 0.02$ and 0.004, respectively).

Sixty-four percent of LEMS patients with SCLC also were found to have antibodies against SOX1, an immunogenic tumor antigen in SCLC. Reports suggest that SOX1 may play a role as an early marker of the future predisposition to LEMS/SCLC.[39] The presence of SOX1 antibodies has a specificity of 95% for SCLC-LEMS; however, sensitivity is only 65%. Titulaer and colleagues[40] have found SOX1 antibodies in fewer than 5% of patients with MG, in up to 25% of patients with lung cancer without LEMS, and in some patients with systemic lupus erythematosus or rheumatoid arthritis who do not have LEMS but have high levels of circulating immunoglobulins. Patients with LEMS with no evidence of cancer at the initial work-up and positive SOX1 antibodies should have close follow-up.

Electrodiagnostic Studies

The classic triad of electrophysiologic findings was first defined by Eaton and Lambert.[3] This triad includes (1) a low CMAP amplitude at rest, (2) a decremental response at low rates of RNS, and (3) an incremental response at high-rate stimulation or after brief exercise (**Fig. 2**). This typical pattern, however, has not been observed in all cases at the time of initial evaluation and a more diverse electrophysiologic spectrum has been described.[41]

The CMAP in LEMS obtained by supramaximal nerve stimulation is often reduced because many muscle fibers are blocked as a result of decreased quantal release of the transmitter.

At slow rates of stimulation (2–3 Hz) a decremental response is seen as additional transmitter depletion occurs. Low-rate RNS shows at least 10% decrement in 94% to 98% of patients with LEMS.[32,42] It has been reported that the decremental pattern with low-rate RNS becomes progressively greater with repeated trains of stimuli in LEMS, whereas in MG, the decrement becomes less pronounced.[43]

After a brief period of voluntary exercise (10–30 seconds), the CMAP in LEMS increases to almost normal size (usually more than double what it was at rest) as a result of calcium facilitation of available transmitter release. There is significantly higher diagnostic sensitivity with the 10-second exercise compared with 30-second exercise at 100% increment and 60% increment levels.[44] Ten seconds of voluntary isometric contraction has a sensitivity of 84% to 96% and is 100% specific for LEMS.[32,44] High-rate stimulation (20–50 Hz) has comparable sensitivity but is painful.[45]

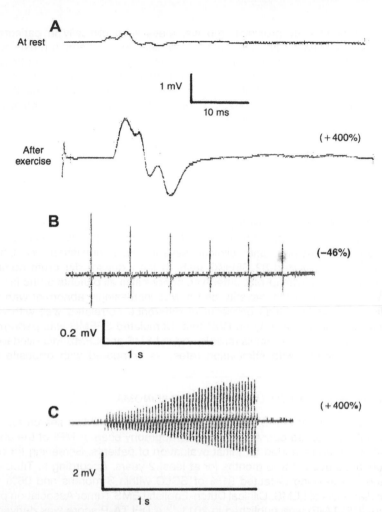

Fig. 2. Typical repetitive nerve stimulation pattern in the abductor digiti minimi muscle in LEMS. (*A*) Low compound action potential amplitude at rest, marked incremental response (+400 mg) after 30 seconds of exercise. (*B*) Decremental response (−46%) at low-rate stimulation (3 Hz). (*C*) Marked incremental response (+400%) at high-rate stimulation (50 Hz). (*From* Oh SJ. Treatment and management of the neuromuscular junction. In: Bertorini TE, editor. Neuromuscular disorders. Treatment and management. Philadelphia: Elsevier-Saunders; 2011. p. 323; with permission.)

High-rate RNS or 10 seconds of voluntary isometric contraction shows the CMAP amplitude immediately increases by greater than 100% in 70% of patients, consistent with a postactivation facilitation.

A cutoff of 60% to consider the CMAP increment significant has been proposed, because it raises sensitivity to 97%, whereas specificity remains 99% in excluding MG.[32] The authors subsequently found that patients with LEMS with positive VGCC antibodies had lower pre-exercise amplitudes and higher postexercise facilitation (meeting a 100% increment as the diagnostic postexercise criterion), whereas all sero-negative cases only met the 60% increment as the diagnostic criterion.[38] In clinical practice, the finding of 100% CMAP amplitude increment after brief exercise provides compelling support for the diagnostic confirmation of LEMS.

Despite predominantly proximal limb weakness seen clinically in patients with LEMS, the characteristic RNS abnormalities are seen in distal and in proximal muscle.[46] In fact, the most sensitive muscles for detecting characteristic electrophysiologic abnormalities of low resting CMAP amplitude and increment of more than 100% after 10 seconds maximal voluntary contraction are abductor digiti minimi, abductor pollicis brevis, and anconeus.[47] Thus, it is usually preferable and adequate enough to do the RNS test on distal muscles, either on the abductor pollicis brevis or abductor digiti minimi muscle.

RNS can be abnormal in other neuromuscular disorders and conventional needle electromyography (EMG) should be considered to exclude a muscle and anterior horn cell diseases. Needle EMG in LEMS demonstrates unstable motor unit action potential.

Single fiber EMG (SFEMG) findings are similar to postsynaptic neuromuscular junction disorders with increased jitter and blocking; however, these findings are frequently out of proportion to the severity of weakness.[48] The relationship between electrodiagnostic findings and clinical severity was published by Oh and colleagues[49] who analyzed 82 SFEMG tests in the extensor digitorum communis muscle in 30 patients with LEMS. Jitter was abnormal in all patients at the first evaluation regardless of clinical severity and it was increasingly abnormal with worsening disease severity. Mean consecutive difference correlated well with clinical and electrophysiologic severity on RNS test. Stimulated SFEMG was performed in the extensor digitorum communis muscle and in LEMS and LEMS/MG overlap, jitter and blocking improve with stimulation rates, as compared with opposite effect in MG.[50]

SCREENING FOR SMALL CELL LUNG CANCER CARCINOMA

When the diagnosis of LEMS has been confirmed, an extensive search for malignancy should be carried out. A computed tomography scan or MRI of the chest or a PET scan is recommended for initial evaluation of patients. Screening for cancer should continue every 3 to 6 months for at least 2 years. According to Titulaer and colleagues,[51] screening detected 91% of SCLC within 3 months and 96% within 1 year of diagnosis of LEMS. Clinical Dutch-English LEMS Tumor Association prediction score (DELTA-P) was published in 2011.[10] A DELTA-P score was derived allocating one point for the presence of each of the following items at or within 3 months from onset: age at onset greater than or equal to 50 years, smoking at diagnosis, weight loss greater than or equal to 5%, bulbar involvement, erectile dysfunction, and Karnofsky performance status lower than 70. The probability for SCLC is calculated at diagnosis of LEMS, and varies from 0.2% to 6% with a DELTA-P score of 0 to 1, up to 83.9% to 100% with a score of 3 to 6. Titulaer and colleagues proposed a screening strategy with computed tomography thorax and F-fluorodeoxyglucose-PET based on a DELTA-P score. In patients with a DELTA-P score of 0 or 1, it was suggested that screening be discontinued after two adequate and negative screens 6 months apart (the chance of SCLC is lower than 1 per 1000). If the score is 2, screening should continue every 6 months for 2 years. If the score is 3 to 6, the second screening should be performed after 3 months and it should be repeated every 6 months afterward for 2 years (**Fig. 3**).

TREATMENT

Treatment of patients with LEMS includes treatment of a tumor when applicable and symptomatic management. AChE inhibitors do not usually produce significant

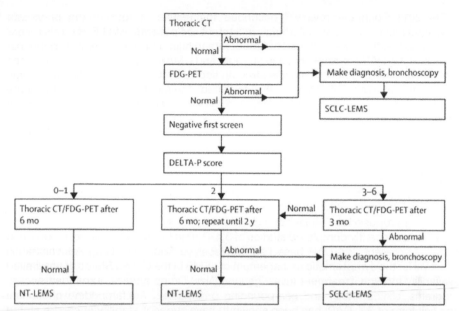

Fig. 3. Flowchart of recommended screening for SCLC in patients with LEMS. CT, computed tomography; FDG, F-fluorodeoxyglucose. (*From* Titulaer MJ, Lang B, Verschuuren JJ. Lambert-Eaton myasthenic syndrome: from clinical characteristics to therapeutic strategies. Lancet Neurol 2011;10(12):1103; Reprinted with permission from Elsevier (The Lancet).)

improvement in LEMS, although they may improve dry mouth. Lambert, in his first report, noted the poor response of his patients to neostigmine.[2] For symptomatic treatment, pyridostigmine, guanidine, 4-aminopyridine, and 3,4-diaminopyridine (3,4-DAP) have been tried.[52,53] Except for 3,4-DAP, these compounds have been studied in small open label case series, but not in clinical trials.

3,4-DAP blocks VGCCs that lead to prolongation of depolarization of the action potential at motor nerve terminals and increase the open time of the VGCCs.[54] This process results in increased presynaptic influx of calcium and enhancement of ACh release manifesting by improvement in muscle function. Typical dosage of prescribed 3,4-DAP is 10 mg by mouth three times a day. Maximum recommended dosage is 80 mg a day.

McEvoy and colleagues[55] in 1989 studied oral 3,4-DAP in a double-blind, randomized, crossover controlled trial in 12 patients with LEMS, seven of whom had cancer. Results of this trial showed significant improvement in neurologic disability score, isometric myometry limb testing strength measures, CMAP amplitude change, and autonomic function change following oral administration of up to 100 mg per day 3,4-DAP compared with the placebo. One patient had a seizure after 10 months of treatment. Another randomized, double-blind, crossover trial of oral 3,4-DAP of up to 80 mg per day showed significant efficacy over the placebo in seven patients with LEMS.[56] Results of the parallel group trial of 26 cases by Sanders and colleagues[57] showed similar results, namely significant improvement of the Quantitative Myasthenia Gravis (QMG) score and resting amplitude following the oral administration of 60 mg per day 3,4-DAP.

Intravenous administration of 3,4-DAP produced similar results. Wirtz and colleagues[58] reported no additional benefit with the addition of pyridostigmine, and pyridostigmine in isolation showed no difference to the placebo group.

The 2011 Cochrane review[59] described the results of four of the previously described randomized controlled trials in a total of 54 patients with LEMS. This review concluded that there was "limited but moderate to high quality evidence showing that over days 3,4-DAP improved muscle strength and CMAP in LEMS." All trials reported a significant improvement in muscle strength score, QMG score, or CMAP amplitude after treatment. Also, 3,4-DAP was well tolerated. The most common side effects are perioral tingling, digital paresthesias, and gastrointestinal symptoms. The most serious adverse events are dose-dependent. Seizures were described at doses of more than 100 mg per day and supraventricular tachycardia with iatrogenic intoxication of 360 mg. Prolongation of the QT interval is often mentioned as a possible side effect.

3,4-DAP was first approved for use in Europe for patients with LEMS in December 2009. It has been recommended as a first-line symptomatic treatment of LEMS by the European Federation of Neurologic Societies since 2010. An algorithm for treatment of LEMS was proposed by Titulaer and coworkers (**Fig. 4**).[21]

Of the two recently completed studies of 3,4-DAP in LEMS, one has been published so far. At present, 3,4-DAP base has not received Food and Drug Administration approval for the symptomatic management of LEMS in the United States. It has limited availability through Treatment Investigational New Drugs studies, expanded-access programs, clinical trials, and compounding pharmacies. Amifampridine phosphate (the salt form of 3,4-DAP) has been shown to have superior stability (it can be stored

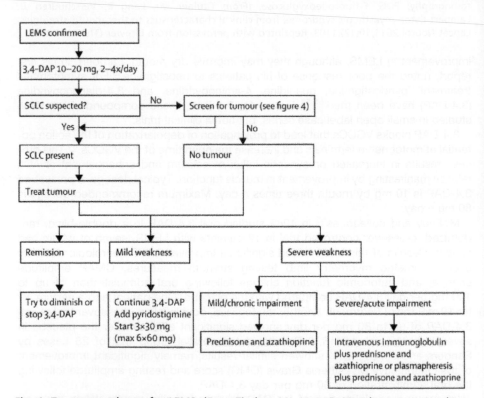

Fig. 4. Treatment scheme for LEMS. (*From* Titulaer MJ, Lang B, Verschuuren JJ. Lambert-Eaton myasthenic syndrome: from clinical characteristics to therapeutic strategies. Lancet Neurol 2011;10(12):1104; Reprinted with permission from Elsevier (The Lancet).)

at room temperature) compared with the base.[60] An oral formulation containing amifampridine phosphate, equivalent to 10 mg base, has been developed (Firdapse, Catalyst Pharmaceuticals, Coral Gables, FL). Amifampridine phosphate has received orphan drug designation and has been granted a Breakthrough Therapy designation by the Food and Drug Administration in 2013.

A phase 3 clinical trial evaluated the efficacy and safety of amifampridine phosphate for symptomatic treatment of LEMS.[61] A multicenter, randomized phase 3 "withdrawal trial" was conducted at 18 sites in the United States, the European Union, and the Russian Federation. Total daily dose of amifampridine phosphate was 15 to 80 mg/d, given in 3 to 4 divided doses, with a maximum single dose of 20 mg. Thirty-eight patients were randomized and the efficacy of amifapridine phosphate at Day 8 and Day 14 was evaluated. The coprimary efficacy end points were the change from baseline to Day 14 in Quantitative Myasthenia Gravis score and in the Subject Global Impression of change. Secondary end points included the changes from baseline in Clinical Global Impression of Improvement and Timed 25-foot-walk-test speed at Day 14. Tertiary end point was the CMAP in the abductor digiti minimi muscle at rest with a single maximal stimulation of the ulnar nerve at the wrist. The primary efficacy end points and one (Clinical Global Impression of Improvement) of the secondary efficacy end points were met, showing a significant benefit of amifampridine phosphate over the placebo at Day 14. Amifampridine phosphate was well tolerated. The most common adverse events were oral (40%) and digital (34%) paresthesias, nausea, and headache. One limitation of this trial is that the protocol was not followed by 10 patients. This study provided class I evidence of efficacy of amifampridine phosphate as a symptomatic treatment of LEMS.

For rapidly progressive LEMS symptoms, intravenous immunoglobulin (IVIG) has been used. A single randomized double-blind, placebo-controlled, crossover study involving patients with LEMS with no carcinoma showed a significant improvement in limb strength (measured by myometry) peaking at 2 to 4 weeks and effects lasting up to 8 weeks following IVIG treatment (1 g/kg body weight/day for 2 days). The clinical response was associated with a significant decline in antibody titer to VGCC.[62] Aside from this trial, there are few data regarding the use of IVIG treatment of LEMS. Experience from case reports indicates that IVIG is useful in patients with LEMS, as a short- and long-term repeated treatment, especially when immunosuppressive drugs are not fully effective.[63–65]

For patients with severe symptoms requiring a prompt management, plasma exchange delivered as a 5-day course, removing 3 to 4 L each day, typically improves LEMS symptoms in cancer and noncancer LEMS. Objective CMAP amplitude outcome measures corresponded to clinical improvement. The peak beneficial effect is usually demonstrated after about 2 weeks, subsiding after 6 weeks.[66]

In patients whose LEMS symptoms are not adequately controlled on symptomatic treatment, long-term oral immunosuppression with prednisolone and azathioprine is usually considered,[67] with treatment regimens based on previous trial data in MG (prednisolone dose is up to 1.5 mg/kg on alternate days; azathioprine a total dose of 2.5 mg/kg per day) showing beneficial effects from combined therapy. The effectiveness of the combined prednisone-azathioprine therapy has only been shown in a retrospective study and part prospective study.[68] Observational follow-up data on 47 patients with NT-LEMS in one center demonstrated that combination therapy of prednisolone and azathioprine was required in proximately 90% patients, with 43% achieving sustained clinical remission within the first 3 years of treatment. However, prednisolone (mean, 30 mg on alternate days, often combined with azathioprine) was still required after 3-year follow-up, with only 14% achieving clinical and pharmacologic remission.

Similar data with modest benefit of prednisone and azathioprine were published from other centers.[69] Observational studies on 73 patients with LEMS (42% with lung cancer) have previously demonstrated that high-dose prednisolone often achieved only mild to moderate improvement in symptoms, which was not sustained when the dose was reduced.[52]

There are isolated reports of medium-term benefit from rituximab[70] and favorable response to rituximab.[71,72] There is a theoretic concern that immunosuppression may reduce the immunologic suppression of tumor growth. Aggressive immunotherapy is more commonly prescribed in patients without cancer. The specific treatment of the underlying tumor usually ultimately results in improvement or even remission of symptoms but symptomatic treatment early on is extremely important for patients to regain and maintain strength and function.

Unlike other paraneoplastic syndromes, which are usually resistant to any therapy, LEMS is known to be consistently responsive to immunotherapy or anticancer therapy.[73] Thus, in patients with the paraneoplastic form of LEMS, it is critical that antitumor treatments are given to treat underlying malignancies. Clinical data suggest that the immune response associated with LEMS may suppress tumor activity, thus prolonging survival times of LEMS patients with cancer.[13,74] This was confirmed in a recent prospective study of 31 LEMS patients with SCLC who were compared with 279 SCLC without neurologic illness. After controlling for known SCLC prognostic factors, the presence of LEMS with SCLC conferred a significant survival advantage, thereby excluding lead time bias as a potential alternate explanation.[75] Chemotherapeutic agents, such as vincristine, doxorubicin, and cyclophosphamide, are effective against SCLC-associated LEMS, but the proportions of patients benefiting are small. In a study of 16 patients with LEMS associated with small cell carcinoma, 13 patients received specific tumor therapy and most also received pharmacologic and immunologic treatment of LEMS.[73]

Seven of 11 patients surviving for more than 2 months after tumor therapy showed substantial neurologic improvement, but only one patient was in complete remission 7 years after the cancer therapy. In 3 of these 11 patients, improvement was only transient.

SUMMARY

LEMS is a rare and unique autoimmune calcium channelopathy. An underlying small cancer is found in more than half of patients with LEMS. Continued cancer screening is required every 3 to 6 months for at least 2 years following symptom onset. Proximal muscle weakness, autonomic features, and areflexia are a typical clinical triad. Characteristic electrophysiologic findings include reduced CMAP amplitudes; decremental response at low-rate RNS; and most importantly an incremental response immediately following 10 seconds of maximal voluntary contraction or in severely weak cases, brief 50 Hz RNS. 3,4-DAP dosed at 30 to 80 mg daily is the most effective symptomatic treatment of LEMS with good tolerability and safety profile.

REFERENCES

1. Anderson HJ, Churchill-Davidson HC, Richardson AT. Bronchial neoplasm with myasthenia: prolonged apnea after administration of succinylcholine. Lancet 1953;265:1291–3.
2. Lambert EH, Eaton LM, Rooke ED. Defect of neuromuscular conduction associated with malignant neoplasms. Am J Physiol 1956;187:612–3.

3. Eaton LM, Lambert EH. Electromyography and electrical stimulation of nerves in diseases of the motor unit: observations on a myasthenic syndrome associated with malignant tumours. J Am Med Assoc 1957;163:1117–24.

4. Rooke ED, Eaton LM, Lambert EH, et al. Myasthenia and malignant intrathoracic tumor. Med Clin North Am 1960;44:977–88.

5. Lambert EH, Rooke ED. Myasthenic state and lung cancer. In: Brain WR, Norris FH Jr, editors. The remote effect of cancer on the nervous system. New York: Grune&Stratton; 1965. p. 67–80.

6. Fukunaga H, Engel AG, Lang B, et al. Paucity and disorganization of presynaptic membrane active zones in the Lambert–Eaton myasthenic syndrome. Muscle Nerve 1982;5:686–97.

7. Lennon VA, Kryzer TJ, Griesmann GE, et al. Calcium-channel antibodies in the Lambert-Eaton syndrome and other paraneoplastic syndromes. N Engl J Med 1995;332:1467–74.

8. Wirtz PW, Nijnuis MG, Sotodeh M, et al. Dutch Myasthenia Study Group. The epidemiology of myasthenia gravis, Lambert-Eaton myasthenic syndrome and their associated tumours in the northern part of the province of South Holland. J Neurol 2003;250(6):698–701.

9. Sanders DB. Lambert-Eaton myasthenic syndrome: diagnosis and treatment. Ann N Y Acad Sci 2003;998:500–8.

10. Titulaer MJ, Maddison P, Sont JK, et al. Clinical Dutch-English Lambert-Eaton myasthenic syndrome (LEMS) tumor association prediction score accurately predicts small-cell lung cancer in the LEMS. J Clin Oncol 2011;29:902–8.

11. Wirtz PW, Smallegange TM, Wintzen AR, et al. Differences in clinical features between the Lambert-Eaton myasthenic syndrome with and without cancer: an analysis of 227 published cases. Clin Neurol Neurosurg 2002;104:359–63.

12. Wirtz PW, Willcox N, van der Slik AR, et al. HLA and smoking in prediction and prognosis of small cell lung cancer in autoimmune Lambert-Eaton myasthenic syndrome. J Neuroimmunol 2005;159:230–7.

13. Titulaer MJ, Verschuuren JJ. Lambert-Eaton myasthenic syndrome: tumor versus nontumor forms. Ann NY Acad Sci 2008;1132:129–34.

14. O'Neill JH, Murray NMF, Newsom-Davis J. The Lambert-Eaton myasthenic syndrome: a review of 50 cases. Brain 1988;111:577–96.

15. Meriney SD, Hulsizer SC, Lennon VA, et al. Lambert-Eaton myasthenic syndrome immunoglobulins react with multiple types of calcium channels in small-cell lung carcinoma. Ann Neurol 1996;40:739–49.

16. Oguro-Okano M, Griesmann GE, Wieben ED, et al. Molecular diversity of neuronal-type calcium channels identified in small cell lung carcinoma. Mayo Clin Proc 1992;67:1150–9.

17. Zalewski NL, Lennon VA, Lachance DH, et al. P/Q- and N-type calcium-channel antibodies: oncological, neurological, and serological accompaniments. Muscle Nerve 2016;54(2):220–7.

18. Katz E, Ferro PA, Weiss G, et al. Calcium channels involved in synaptic transmission at the mature and regenerating mouse neuromuscular junction. J Physiol 1996;497:687–9.

19. Hirning LD, Fox AP, McCleskey EW, et al. Dominant role of N-type Ca21 channels in evoked release of norepinephrine from sympathetic neurons. Science 1998;239:57–61.

20. Lang B, Newsom-Davis J, Wray D, et al. Autoimmune etiology for myasthenic (Eaton-Lambert) syndrome. Lancet 1981;2:224–6.

21. Titulaer MJ, Lang B, Verschuuren JJ. Lambert-Eaton myasthenic syndrome: from clinical characteristics to therapeutic strategies. Lancet Neurol 2011;10(12): 1098–107.

22. Titulaer MJ, Wirtz PW, Kuks JB, et al. The Lambert-Eaton myasthenic syndrome 1988–2008: a clinical picture in 97 patients. J Neuroimmunol 2008;201–02:153–8.

23. Burns TM, Russell JA, LaChance DH, et al. Oculobulbar involvement is typical with Lambert-Eaton myasthenic syndrome. Ann Neurol 2003;53:270–3.

24. Young JD, Leavitt JA. Lambert Eaton myasthenic syndrome: ocular signs and symptoms. J Neuroophthalmol 2016;36:20–2.

25. Oh SJ. The Eaton-Lambert syndrome in ocular myasthenia gravis. Arch Neurol 1974;31:183–6.

26. Rudnicki SA. Lambert-Eaton myasthenic syndrome with pure ocular weakness. Neurology 2007;68:1863–4.

27. Smith AG, Wald J. Acute ventilatory failure in Lambert-Eaton myasthenic syndrome and its response to 3,4-diaminopyridine. Neurology 1996;46:1143–5.

28. Lorenzoni PJ, Scola RH, Kay CS, et al. Non-paraneoplastic Lambert-Eaton myasthenic syndrome: a brief review of 10 cases. Arq Neuropsiquiatr 2010;68:849–54.

29. Pellkofer HL, Armbruster L, Linke R, et al. Managing non-paraneoplastic Lambert-Eaton myasthenic syndrome: clinical characteristics in 25 German patients. J Neuroimmunol 2009;217:90–4.

30. Waterman SA, Lang B, Newsom-Davis J. Effect of Lambert-Eaton myasthenic syndrome antibodies on autonomic neurons in the mouse. Ann Neurol 1997;42: 147–56.

31. Khurana RK, Koski CL, Mayer RF. Autonomic dysfunction in Lambert-Eaton myasthenic syndrome. J Neurol Sci 1988;85:77–86.

32. Oh SJ, Kurokawa K, Claussen GC, et al. Electrophysiological diagnostic criteria of Lambert-Eaton myasthenic syndrome. Muscle Nerve 2005;32:515–20.

33. Odabasi Z, Demirci M, Kim DS, et al. Postexercise facilitation of reflexes is not common in Lambert-Eaton myasthenic syndrome. Neurology 2002;59:1085–7.

34. Oh SJ. Myasthenia gravis Lambert-Eaton overlap syndrome. Muscle Nerve 2016; 53:20–6.

35. Motomura M, Lang B, Johnston I, et al. Incidence of serum anti-P/Q-type and anti-N-type calcium channel autoantibodies in the Lambert-Eaton myasthenic syndrome. J Neurol Sci 1997;147;35–42.

36. Hajela RK, Huntoon KM, Atchison WD. Lambert-Eaton syndrome antibodies target multiple subunits of voltage-gated Ca2+ channels. Muscle Nerve 2015; 51(2):176–84.

37. Nakao YK, Motomura M, Fukudome T, et al. Seronegative Lambert-Eaton myasthenic syndrome. Neurology 2002;59:1773–5.

38. Oh SJ, Hatanaka Y, Claussen GC, et al. Electrophysiological differences in seropositive and seronegative Lambert-Eaton myasthenic syndrome. Muscle Nerve 2007;35:178–83.

39. Sabater L, Titulaer M, Saiz A, et al. SOX1 antibodies are markers of paraneoplastic Lambert–Eaton myasthenic syndrome. Neurology 2008;70:924–8.

40. Titulaer MJ, Klooster R, Potman M, et al. SOX antibodies in small-cell lung cancer and Lambert-Eaton myasthenic syndrome: frequency and relation with survival. J Clin Oncol 2009;27:4260–7.

41. Oh SJ. Diverse electrophysiological spectrum of the Lambert-Eaton myasthenic syndrome. Muscle Nerve 1989;12:464–9.

42. Tim RW, Massey JM, Sanders DB. Lambert-Eaton myasthenic syndrome (LEMS): clinical and electrodiagnostic features and response to therapy in 59 patients. Ann N Y Acad Sci 1998;841:823–6.

43. Sanders DB, Cao L, Massey JM, et al. Is the decremental pattern in Lambert-Eaton syndrome different from that in myasthenia gravis? Clin Neurophysiol 2014;125(6):1274–7.

44. Hatanaka Y, Oh SJ. Ten-second exercise is superior to 30-second exercise for post-exercise facilitation in diagnosing Lambert-Eaton myasthenic syndrome. Muscle Nerve 2008;37:572–5.

45. Tim RW, Sanders DB. Repetitive nerve stimulation studies in the Lambert-Eaton myasthenic syndrome. Muscle Nerve 1994;17(9):995–1001.

46. Oh SJ. Electromyography: neuromuscular transmission studies. Baltimore (MD): Williams & Wilkins; 1988.

47. Maddison P, Newsom-Davis J, Mills KR. Distribution of electrophysiological abnormality in Lambert-Eaton myasthenic syndrome. J Neurol Neurosurg Psychiatry 1998;65:213–7.

48. Sanders DB, Stålberg EV. AAEM minimonograph #25: single-fiber electromyography. Muscle Nerve 1996;19:1069–83.

49. Oh SJ, Ohira M. Single-fiber EMG and clinical correlation in Lambert-Eaton myasthenic syndrome. Muscle Nerve 2013;47(5):664–7.

50. Chaudhry V, Watson DF, Bird SJ, et al. Stimulated single-fiber electromyography in Lambert-Eaton myasthenic syndrome. Muscle Nerve 1991;14(12):1227–30.

51. Titulaer MJ, Wirtz PW, Willems LN, et al. Screening for small-cell lung cancer: a follow-up study of patients with Lambert-Eaton myasthenic syndrome. J Clin Oncol 2008;26:4276–81.

52. Tim RW, Massey JM, Sanders DB. Lambert-Eaton myasthenic syndrome: electrodiagnostic finding and response to treatment. Neurology 2000;54:2176–8.

53. Oh SJ, Kim DS, Head TC, et al. Low-dose guanidine and pyridostigmine: relatively safe and effective long-term symptomatic therapy in Lambert-Eaton myasthenic syndrome. Muscle Nerve 1997;20:1146–52.

54. Molgo J, Lundh H, Thesle S. Potency of 3,4-diaminopyridine and 4-aminopyridine on mammalian neuromuscular transmission and the effect of pH changes. Eur J Pharmacol 1980;61:25–34.

55. McEvoy KM, Windebank AJ, Daube JR, et al. 3,4-Diaminopyridine in the treatment of Lambert-Eaton myasthenic syndrome. N Engl J Med 1989;321:1567–71.

56. Oh SJ, Claussen GG, Hatanaka Y, et al. 3,4-Diaminopyridine is more effective than placebo in a randomized, double-blind, cross-over drug study in LEMS. Muscle Nerve 2009;40:795–800.

57. Sanders DB, Massey JM, Sanders LL, et al. A randomized trial of 3,4-diaminopyridine in Lambert-Eaton myasthenic syndrome. Neurology 2000;54(3):603–7.

58. Wirtz PW, Verschuuren JJ, van Dijk JG, et al. Efficacy of 3,4-diaminopyridine and pyridostigmine in the treatment of Lambert-Eaton myasthenic syndrome: a randomized, double-blind, placebo-controlled, crossover study. Clin Pharmacol Ther 2009;86(1):44–8.

59. Keogh M, Sedehizadeh S, Maddison P. Treatment for Lambert-Eaton myasthenic syndrome. Cochrane Database Syst Rev 2011;(2):CD003279.

60. Raust JA, Goulay-Dufay S, Le Hoang MD, et al. Stability studies of ionised and non-ionised 3,4-diaminopyridine: hypothesis of degradation pathways and chemical structure of degradation products. J Pharm Biomed Anal 2007;43:83–8.

61. Oh SJ, Shcherbakova N, Kostera-Pruszczyk A, et al. Amifampridine phosphate (Firdapse(®)) is effective and safe in a phase 3 clinical trial in LEMS. Muscle Nerve 2016;53(5):717–25.

62. Bain PG, Motomura M, Newsom-Davis J, et al. Effects of intravenous immuno-globulin on muscle weakness and calcium-channel autoantibodies in the Lambert-Eaton myasthenic syndrome. Neurology 1996;47:678–83.

63. Illa I. IVIg in myasthenia gravis, Lambert Eaton myasthenic syndrome and inflammatory myopathies: current status. J Neurol 2005;252(Suppl 1):I14–8.

64. Muchnik S, Losavio AS, Vidal A, et al. Long-term follow-up of Lambert-Eaton syndrome treated with intravenous immunoglobulin. Muscle Nerve 1997;20(6):674–8.

65. Bird SJ. Clinical and electrophysiologic improvement in Lambert-Eaton syndrome with intravenous immunoglobulin therapy. Neurology 1992;42:1422–3.

66. Newsom-Davis J, Murray NM. Plasma exchange and immunosuppressive drug treatment in the Lambert-Eaton myasthenic syndrome. Neurology 1984;34:480–5.

67. Newsom-Davis J. A treatment algorithm for Lambert-Eaton myasthenic syndrome. Ann NY Acad Sci 1998;841:817–22.

68. Maddison P, Lang B, Mills K, et al. Long term outcome in Lambert-Eaton myasthenic syndrome without lung cancer. J Neurol Neurosurg Psychiatry 2001; 70(2):212–7.

69. Maddison P. Treatment in Lambert-Eaton myasthenic syndrome. Ann N Y Acad Sci 2012;1275:78–84.

70. Maddison P, McConville J, Farrugia ME, et al. The use of rituximab in myasthenia gravis and Lambert-Eaton myasthenic syndrome. J Neurol Neurosurg Psychiatry 2011;82(6):671–3.

71. Pellkofer HL, Voltz R, Kuempfel T. Favorable response to rituximab in a patient with anti-VGCC-positive Lambert-Eaton myasthenic syndrome and cerebellar dysfunction. Muscle Nerve 2009;40(2):305–8.

72. Boutin E, Rey C, Romeu M, et al. Favourable outcome after treatment with rituximab in a case of seronegative non-paraneoplastic Lambert-Eaton myasthenic syndrome. Rev Med Interne 2013;34(8):493–6.

73. Chalk CH, Murray NM, Newsome-Davis J, et al. Responses of the Lambert-Eason myasthenic syndrome to treatment of associated small-cell lung cancer. Neurology 1990;40:1552–6.

74. Maddisson P, Newsome-Davis J, Mills KR, et al. Favorable prognosis in Lambert-Eaton myasthenic syndrome and small-cell lung carcinoma. Lancet 1999;353: 117–8.

75. Maddison P, Gozzard P, Grainge MJ, et al. Long-term survival in paraneoplastic Lambert-Eaton myasthenic syndrome. Neurology 2017;88(14):1334–9.

Moving?

Make sure your subscription moves with you!

To notify us of your new address, find your **Clinics Account Number** (located on your mailing label above your name), and contact customer service at:

Email: journalscustomerservice-usa@elsevier.com

800-654-2452 (subscribers in the U.S. & Canada)
314-447-8871 (subscribers outside of the U.S. & Canada)

Fax number: 314-447-8029

Elsevier Health Sciences Division
Subscription Customer Service
3251 Riverport Lane
Maryland Heights, MO 63043

*To ensure uninterrupted delivery of your subscription, please notify us at least 4 weeks in advance of move.

Printed and bound by CPI Group (UK) Ltd, Croydon, CR0 4YY

07/10/2024

01040504-0013